Study Guide for Huber
Leadership and Nursing Care Management

Jean Nagelkerk, RN, PhD
Associate Professor of Nursing
Grand Valley State University
Grand Rapids, Michigan

W.B. Saunders Company
A Division of Harcourt Brace & Company
Philadelphia   London   Toronto   Montreal   Sydney   Tokyo

W. B. SAUNDERS COMPANY
A Division of Harcourt Brace & Company

The Curtis Center
Independence Square West
Philadelphia, Pennsylvania 19106

Study Guide for Huber:
Leadership and Nursing Care Management   0–7216–6819–4

Printed in the United States of America

Last digit is the print number: 9   8   7   6   5   4   3   2   1

Table of Contents

PART V   MANAGING PROFESSIONALS AND THEIR PRACTICE

PART VI   EVALUATION AND CONTROL IN NURSING ADMINISTRATION

Chapter 1

Overview of Nursing Administration

STUDY FOCUS

Nursing administration is very important in providing quality healthcare to communities. Nursing administration is the act of synthesizing management theory and nursing practice, using power and authority to provide quality care, and managing the healthcare delivery system to meet the community-based needs of clients. Nursing administration theory and knowledge is derived from three primary sources: nursing, management, and leadership theory. Theory and concepts are also drawn from other sources such as anthropology, education, psychology, sociology, and public health. Integrating nursing knowledge and knowledge from a combination of disciplines enables nurses to gain new insights into clinical and administrative practice.

Nursing administration is complex and involves using different categories of nurses to provide quality healthcare to clients. Nurse executives provide leadership by developing strategic plans, implementing new programs, and coordinating the delivery of nursing services to clients. Nurse executives look at the "big picture" and make long-range decisions for the organization. Nurse managers help nurse executives by working on day-to-day management activities and coordinating nursing care at the unit level. Nurse care providers are integral to coordinating and providing direct care to clients. These three categories of individuals work as a team to provide the best care possible.

All categories of nurses use leadership and management behaviors to accomplish their work. Leadership focuses on influencing people to accomplish goals, inspiring confidence, envisioning the future, and motivating followers by leading the way. Management, on the other hand, coordinates and integrates resources, plans, organizes, directs, controls, and accomplishes organizational goals. Leadership and management overlap by focusing on goal accomplishment and motivating and directing followers. The most effective nurses use both leadership and management behaviors to accomplish their goals and motivate other nurses and clients.

LEARNING TOOLS

Group Activity: Understanding Nursing Administration

Purpose: To help you understand how different disciplines enhance the practice of nursing, and to enable you to discuss the interdependence of nursing with other disciplines. The disciplines that will be explored are nursing, management, business, education, and psychology.

Divide the study group into five groups.

Assign each group to either nursing, management, business, education, or psychology.

Each small group should take 20 minutes to identify material that is important for nursing administration. For example, one important item from business may be how to work with budgets. Effective nurse administrators must be knowledgeable about the costs of providing care to clients.

When 20 minutes are up, one member from each group should make a verbal report to the study group on how the assigned discipline influences nursing care.

The study group leader should summarize the discussion.

CASE STUDY

June Hill, R.N., works as a care provider on 3 East, a neurological unit at Western Hospital. June works in a case management system and coordinates care for a case load of clients, interacting with physicians, nurses, other healthcare workers, and outside agencies. She is viewed by her peers as a resource and is constantly sought for advice. June established the care management system on her unit, motivated her peers to "buy into" the new system, and convinced her manager that it was worthwhile. She enjoys her work and is continually influencing others to meet the goals she sets for client care.

Case Study Questions

1. Is June exhibiting leadership or management behaviors?

[handwritten annotations: coordinates care, case management system, interacting c̄ physicians; Influencing, resource sought for advice]

2. Can a nurse in a care provider position lead and/ or manage? _Both_
3. What behaviors make a nurse an effective leader?
4. What behaviors make a nurse an effective manager?

LEARNING RESOURCES

Discussion Questions

1. How can nurses use information from other disciplines to enhance their practice?
2. What is nursing administration, and what is the role of a practicing nurse in the provision and delivery of high quality patient care?
3. How do leadership and management differ? Is it useful to possess both leadership and management behaviors?
4. Are all nurses in organizations involved in nursing administration? In what way?
5. What is the difference between a nurse executive, a nurse manager, and a nurse care provider?

Study Questions

True and False: Circle the correct answer.

(T) F 1. In acute care, the traditional medical model is predominant.

(T) F 2. The two basic roles of clinical nurses are to provide direct care and to supervise the care of clients.

T (F) 3. Conceptual acts include thinking, making decisions, and implementing plans.

(T) F 4. Nursing administration is the combination of leadership and management knowledge applied to nursing care delivery.

T (F) 5. Leadership and management are distinct ideas with no overlap.

T (F) 6. The two most common disciplines nurse managers synthesize are nursing and physiology.

T (F) 7. Nurse managers should not be concerned with organizational finances; they should focus on client care.

(T) F 8. The most effective nurses use a combination of leadership and management behaviors.

T (F) 9. Leadership is the coordination and integration of resources and plans to accomplish organizational objectives. _Management_

T (F) 10. Management is influencing people to accomplish goals and motivating followers by leading the way.

SUPPLEMENTAL READINGS

Henry, B., Arndt, C., Vincenti, M.D. & Marriner-Tomey, A. (1989). _Dimensions of Nursing Administration._ Blackwell Scientific Publication.

Smith, M.C. (1993). The contribution of nursing theory to nursing administration practice. _Image: Journal of Nursing Scholarship_ 25(1), 63-67.

Chapter 2

The Healthcare System

STUDY FOCUS

Understanding the healthcare system is important for providing high quality care at a reasonable cost to consumers. A healthcare system is composed of structures, organizations, and services designed to deliver professional health services to consumers. Integrated healthcare systems are formed in an attempt to increase efficiency and decrease cost by organizing a collection of healthcare providers to work interdependently and function as an open system which adapts quickly to changes. All healthcare systems consist of five major components: production of resources, organizational structure, management, economic support, and delivery of services (Roemer, 1986). The five leading types of healthcare organizations are hospitals and other acute care institutions, ambulatory care, long-term care facilities, home health agencies, and mental health facilities (Kovner, 1990).

Healthcare systems are being held accountable for the cost of services which provide quality care to clients. In the past, healthcare providers charged fixed fees for services provided. Today, prospective payment systems such as diagnostic related groupings are in place to limit and reduce costs for Medicare clients in hospitals. The federal government funds two major programs—Medicare and Medicaid. Medicare is a two-part program of assistance with healthcare costs for individuals over 65 years of age and those who are disabled. Medicare Part A covers hospital costs and some nursing home care, and Part B covers physician services. Medicaid is a joint federal and state program, administered by the states, to pay for indigents' healthcare.

Despite efforts to contain costs, the total healthcare expenditures continue to rise at an alarming rate. The three categories of greatest total expenditure for healthcare are hospital care, physician fees, and prescription drugs. Widespread concern exists that healthcare expenditures will continue to climb as the number of older citizens and of cases of chronic illnesses increase. Changing ethnicity patterns, accelerating use of high technology, and escalating numbers of those infected with AIDS are also factors. Nurses will be challenged to provide community based care to all clients, to contain costs, and to provide high quality care.

LEARNING TOOLS

Group Activity: Understanding Healthcare Systems

Purpose: To help you understand the U.S. healthcare system and to describe the impact of economics and governmental regulation on healthcare. The cost of healthcare in the U.S., the methods of controlling costs through integrated healthcare systems, and nursing's role in a changing healthcare environment will be examined.

Divide the study group into three groups.

Assign each group to one of these topics: Cost of healthcare in the U.S., methods of controlling costs through integrated healthcare systems, or nursing's role in providing access to care for clients, containing costs, and ensuring high quality care.

Each group should identify important points for the assigned topic (refer to the Huber text Chapter 2 for base information).

Provide 25 minutes for group discussion, and then have each group summarize its recommendations for large group discussion.

The study group leaders should serve as facilitators and summarize information.

CASE STUDY

Healthcare has become a big business in the United States and is very competitive in providing cost-effective care to clients. Stiff competition for market share and costs are being weighed carefully before services are provided. Nurses are now in a position where they are expected not only to provide high quality care at reasonable costs, but also to make recommendations that decrease costs while maintaining exemplary client care. Many factors influence the cost of healthcare for individuals. The three categories with the highest total expenditures include hospital costs, physician fees, and prescription drugs. Other factors that influence costs are extensive. The aging population, changing ethnicity patterns, and the increasing incidence of chronic illness, as well as government regulation and administrative costs for insurance handling; the lack of practice standardization and defensive medicine; the overcapacity of hospital beds; consumer expectations and the lack of healthy lifestyle practices; and new diseases and treatment contribute to rising costs.

Case Study Questions

1. How can nurses impact the cost of client care without compromising quality?
2. What strategies can nurses use to improve client care outcomes?
3. What cost factors do nurses control? What cost factors do nurses have influence over?
4. What could happen to the profession of nursing if nurses elect to ignore cost factors?

LEARNING RESOURCES

Discussion Questions

1. Can the five leading types of healthcare organizations (acute care, ambulatory care, long-term care, home health, and mental health facilities) form an integrated healthcare system? What are the advantages or disadvantages of integrated healthcare systems?
2. What is Medicare? What is Medicaid?
3. Healthcare expenditures continue to rise. What will happen to U.S. businesses if health insurance benefits continue to escalate in cost?
4. Are nursing positions "safe" from downsizing and reductions in staff as healthcare agencies continue to cut costs? What strategies should nurses use to show their impact on patient outcomes?
5. How will nursing's role change as acute care agencies decrease in size and number, and community-based care increases?

Study Questions

Matching: Write the letter of the correct response in front of each term.

<u>D</u>   1. Healthcare System

<u>E</u>   2. Integrated Healthcare System

<u>B</u>   3. Medicare

<u>C</u>   4. Medicaid

<u>F</u>   5. Diagnostic Related Group

<u>A</u>   6. Prospective Payment System

A. a payment system where prices are set before the service is provided

B. federal government healthcare payment system for the over-65 age individual

C. federal and state healthcare payment program for indigent care

D. structure and services to deliver healthcare to patients

E. multiple healthcare agencies linked together to provide seamless healthcare

F. categories of care based on severity of illness grouped according to medical conditions

True and False: Circle the correct answer.

(T)   F   1. Nurse administrators must balance access, cost, and quality to ensure excellent healthcare.

T   (F)   2. Managed care indicates that one healthcare provider delivers all care to a case load of clients.

(T)   F   3. Frequently, hospital bills contain extra healthcare charges.

T   (F)   4. Nursing care is the highest category in the gross national product of total healthcare expenditures in the United States.

SUPPLEMENTAL READINGS

Koevner, A. (1990). *Health care delivery in the United States* (4th ed.). New York: Springer.

Roemer, M. (1986). *An introduction to the U.S. health care system* (2nd ed). New York: Springer.

Tokarski, C. (1995). A new rhythm for the blues, *Hospitals,* 5(69), 23-26.

Wagner, L. (1995). Entitlements: Can we make a new deal? *Hospitals,* 2(69), 24-28.

Chapter 3

Professional Nursing Practice

STUDY FOCUS

Is nursing a profession or an occupation? A profession is comprised of a system of roles that is socially defined. Professions hold contracts with society to provide services for the public good. In return for these essential services, society affords professionals (one who is engaged in a profession) higher prestige, income, and autonomy in their work. Professionalism is the extent to which an individual identifies with a profession and adheres to its standards. Members of society expect that professionals will uphold society's trust by possessing characteristics of expertise, engaging in rigorous academic preparation, and demonstrating commitment and responsible behavior. Professionalization is the process by which occupations set standards to move from non-professional status to a professional one.

The three most common criteria identified by authors as needed for a profession are service, knowledge, and autonomy. Service is providing society with essential activities; knowledge is the strong base of specialized education from which a profession practices; and professional autonomy is having authority over and accountability for one's decisions and activities. All professions have a code of ethics that guides practice. Professionalization of an occupation can be viewed on a continuum. An occupational group can move along the continuum from non-professional to semi-professional to professional.

Nursing requires a high level of expertise, sophisticated decision making, and a sense of service which are characteristic of professional groups. Problematic areas for nursing have been a lack of differentiated practice (multiple educational levels equated with one job assignment), the historical influence of religion and the military, nurses' own attitudes toward professionalization, and the fact that nursing is a profession in which most workers are women. Strong nursing leadership is required to assist in the professionalization of nursing. Nursing leaders must support autonomous nursing practice (job autonomy), continue to develop a strong nursing knowledge base, and use and contribute to nursing research, while being role models of professional behaviors. Using positive media images, educating the public about nursing's role in healthcare, acting altruistically in policy making, and dressing and acting in a professional manner will also enhance the status and profession of nursing.

LEARNING TOOLS

Self-assessment

Valiga Concept of Nursing Scale

Directions: Through the following statements, I am attempting to ascertain the ideas which you currently hold about nursing as a profession, the role of the nurse, and the relationship of the nurse to the client and to the physician and other health team colleagues. Read each of the statements below carefully. Then for each statement please indicate whether you *Strongly Agree (SA), Agree (A),* are *Undecided or Do Not Know (U), Disagree (D),* or *Strongly Disagree (SD)* with the statement. Circle the *one* response that best expresses your opinion, and please be certain your response to each statement is clearly marked. *There are no right or wrong answers,* so please respond openly and honestly.

1. Nurses must be willing to enter with clients those health-related situations which patients cannot face alone. SA A U D SD

2. Nursing is concerned with helping people maximize their health potential in their particular life situation. SA A U D SD

3. Overt action, directed by logical thought, toward meeting the client's need for help constitutes the practice of clinical nursing. SA A U D SD

4. Nurses must assume responsibility for diagnosing and treating human responses to actual or potential illnesses.　SA　A　U　D　SD

5. The independent functions of nurses include supervising the care of clients, observing and recording, supervising nonprofessional personnel, and health teaching.　SA　A　U　D　SD

6. Nursing must be concerned equally with the prevention of disease and the conservation of health.　SA　A　U　D　SD

7. Nursing is an expression of one's commitment to others.　SA　A　U　D　SD

8. Nurses must be involved actively in professional organizations.　SA　A　U　D　SD

9. There is definitely a right and a wrong way to do things and approach nursing situations.　SA　A　U　D　SD

10. Nurses should make written or verbal contacts with all appropriate persons to assure continuity of nursing care for clients.　SA　A　U　D　SD

11. The uniqueness of nursing lies in the reasons for what nurses do in society, rather than in the specific tasks they perform.　SA　A　U　D　SD

12. Nurses should be concerned primarily with giving physical care to clients as directed by the physician.　SA　A　U　D　SD

13. There should be only one nursing theory.　SA　A　U　D　SD

14. Evaluation of the work of their peers and other nursing personnel should be a responsibility of nurses.　SA　A　U　D　SD

15. Nurses must follow doctor's orders without question.　SA　A　U　D　SD

16. Nurses should be free to practice nursing as they define it within the scope of professional autonomy.　SA　A　U　D　SD

17. Nurses should assume responsibility for the total nursing care of a caseload of clients.　SA　A　U　D　SD

18. Nurses should update their knowledge through lifelong continuing education.　SA　A　U　D　SD

19. Nurses must control and direct their own practice.　SA　A　U　D　SD

20. Nurses should be responsible for conducting nursing care conferences routinely.　SA　A　U　D　SD

21. Nurses must be aware that people who require their assistance are helpless and dependent and usually need to be told what to do.　SA　A　U　D　SD

22. Nurses have a responsibility for discussing the proposed medical plan of care with the physician so it can be adjusted, if possible, to be more acceptable to the client.　SA　A　U　D　SD

23. Nurses must assume responsibility for reviewing and evaluating care provided my nursing peers.　SA　A　U　D　SD

24. Nurses must take deliberate action to attain independence in nursing situations.　SA　A　U　D　SD

25. Nurses must not hesitate to assume the role of leader of the healthcare team when the client's problems are best met by nurses.　SA　A　U　D　SD

Scoring: Each individual receives a score of +2 for each item with which they strongly agree, +1 for each item with which they agree, zero for each item about which they were unsure, -1 for each item with which they disagreed, and -2 for each item with which they strongly disagreed. The minimum score is -50 and the maximum score is +50. The higher the + score, the stronger the professional view.

(Courtesy of Theresa M. Valiga, RN, EdD, Dean and Professor, School of Nursing, Fairfield University, Fairfield, Connecticut)

CASE STUDY

Kay is a staff nurse on the oncology unit at Zimmer Hospital in Austin, Texas. She has been a registered nurse for three years. Kay graduated with a baccalaureate degree in nursing and has continued to enroll in one course per term toward her master's degree. Kay is active in the Texas Nurses Association, and she is the secretary for the local Oncology Nurses Association. She subscribes to two nursing journals and attends continuing educational programs at the hospital. She enjoys her work and volunteers for clinical projects.

Case Study Questions

1. Does Kay demonstrate behaviors that indicate she is career or occupation oriented?
2. What characteristics of a professional nurse does Kay demonstrate?

LEARNING RESOURCES

Discussion Questions

1. What are the categories on the continuum of professionalization? Which category does nursing fit?
2. Does nursing fit the major three categories of a profession (service, knowledge, and autonomy)?
3. How does advanced nursing practice fit into professional nursing practice?
4. What barriers are there in nursing's process of professionalization? What driving forces influence nursing's process of professionalization?
5. How have nursing's historical influences (religion and the military) and gender issues influenced nursing's quest toward professionalization?

Study Questions

Matching: Write the letter of the correct response in front of each term.

G	1. Professionalism	A.	comprised of a system of roles that are socially defined
A	2. Profession		
F	3. Professional	B.	one educational level for one job assignment
H	4. Professionalization		
B	5. Differentiated Practice	C.	the authority and accountability for one's work
E	6. Altruism	D.	individual and collective authority and accountability
C	7. Job Autonomy		
D	8. Professional Autonomy	E.	selfless concern and service to others
		F.	one who is engaged in a profession
		G.	the extent to which an individual identifies and adheres to professional standards
		H.	process where occupations change in the direction of a profession

SUPPLEMENTAL READINGS

Chitty, K.K. (1993). Defining profession. In Chitty, K. (Ed.), *Professional nursing concepts and challenge* (pp. 113-123). Philadelphia: W.B. Saunders.

Chitty, K.K. (1993). Professional socialization. In Chitty, K. (Ed.), *Professional nursing concepts and challenge* (pp. 136-155). Philadelphia: W.B. Saunders.

Chapter 4

Leadership Principles

STUDY FOCUS

Leadership is the process of influencing people to accomplish goals by inspiring confidence and support among followers. Skill at interpersonal relationships and applying the problem-solving process are fundamental to leadership. Strong leadership empowers individuals and instills them with a belief and confidence in their ability to achieve and succeed. In contrast, management is the process of influencing employees to work toward the organization's goals by integrating resources through planning, organizing, coordinating, directing, and controlling.

The five interwoven aspects of leadership are the leader, the follower, the situation, the communication process, and the goals (Kison, 1989). Leaders' values, experiences, skills, and expertise are important ingredients in their ability to lead effectively. Transactional leaders function in a caretaker role focusing on day-to-day operations. Transformational leaders motivate followers to perform to their full potential and provide a sense of direction. Followers either reject or accept the leader and determine their own level of participation and the leader's power within the group. Followers may exhibit the Pygmalion effect; that is, acting according to what the leader expects. The situation includes the work to be done, control systems, available resources, the amount of time, the level of interaction, and the external forces impacting the type of decision task. The communication process is the vital means (or way) for leaders and followers to send and receive clear messages, both verbal and nonverbal, through formal and informal channels. The goals include the organizational, personal, and professional goals of the leader and follower.

Leadership characteristics include taking risks, communicating a vision, empowering the followership, mastering change, and motivating groups to achieve goals. There are many leadership theories including attitudinal leadership, situational leadership, Fiedler's contingency, and Hersey and Blanchard's tridimensional leader effectiveness model. Three styles of leadership are authoritarian, democratic, and laissez-faire. Authoritarian leadership refers to directive and controlling behaviors by which the leader in isolation determines policies and makes decisions, and then orders subordinates to carry out the tasks or work. This style is helpful in crisis situations. Democratic leadership is a team approach whereby the leader facilitates and coordinates material and human resources and shares responsibility for decision making and quality improvement. All members of the group are encouraged to actively participate in a cohesive fashion to accomplish team objectives. The democratic leadership style is useful when professional staff work together to establish and meet goals. A laissez-faire leader is one who does not interfere in decision making or policy setting through preference or incompetence. This style may be useful with highly qualified professionals who work well in teams to accomplish established goals.

Nurse leaders are challenged in today's rapidly changing practice environment. They need to exert effective leadership in order to affect positive organizational and individual productivity. At a national level, nurses, representing the largest healthcare profession in the United States, need to band together to provide leadership and direction in healthcare delivery. Nurses must also provide leadership in advocating positive healthcare practices for clients and communities.

LEARNING TOOLS

Task Orientation and People Orientation Leadership Questionnaire:
An Assessment of Style

Purpose: To assess your leadership style in the areas of task and people orientation and to assess your leadership style profile in relation to autocratic, shared (democratic), and laissez-faire leadership.

Directions: The following items describe aspects of leadership behavior. Respond to each item according to the way you would most likely act if you were the leader of a work group. Circle whether you would most likely behave in the described way: always (A), frequently (F), occasionally (O), seldom (S), or never (N).

A F O S N 1. I would most likely act as the spokesman of the group.

A F O S N 2. I would encourage overtime work.

A F O S N 3. I would allow members complete freedom in their work.

A F O S N 4. I would encourage the use of uniform procedures.

A F O S N 5. I would permit the members to use their own judgment in solving problems.

A F O S N 6. I would stress being ahead of competing groups.

A F O S N 7. I would speak as a representative of the group.

A F O S N 8. I would needle members for greater effort.

A F O S N 9. I would try out my ideas in the group.

A F O S N 10. I would let the members do their work the way they think best.

A F O S N 11. I would be working hard for a promotion.

A F O S N 12. I would tolerate postponement and uncertainty.

A F O S N 13. I would speak for the group if there were visitors present.

A F O S N 14. I would keep the work moving at a rapid pace.

A F O S N 15. I would turn the members loose on a job and let them go to it.

A F O S N 16. I would settle conflicts when they occur in the group.

A F O S N 17. I would get swamped by details.

A F O S N 18. I would represent the group at outside meetings.

A F O S N 19. I would be reluctant to allow the members any freedom of action.

A F O S N 20. I would decide what should be done and how it should be done.

A F O S N 21. I would push for increased production.

A F O S N 22. I would let some members have authority which I could keep.

A F O S N 23. Things would usually turn out as I had predicted.

A F O S N 24. I would allow the group a high degree of initiative.

A F O S N 25. I would assign group members to particular tasks.

A F O S N 26. I would be willing to make changes.

A F O S N 27. I would ask the members to work harder.

A F O S N 28. I would trust the group members to exercise good judgment.

A F O S N 29. I would schedule the work to be done.

A F O S N 30. I would refuse to explain my actions.

A F O S N 31. I would persuade others that my ideas are to their advantage.

A F O S N 32. I would permit the group to set its own pace.

A F O S N 33. I would urge the group to beat its previous record.

A F O S N 34. I would act without consulting the group.

A F O S N 35. I would ask that group members follow standard rules and regulations.

T _____   P _____

Scoring: *First:* Circle the item number for items 8, 12, 17, 18, 19, 30, 34, and 35. Write the number 1 in front of a circled item number if you responded S (seldom) or N (never) to that item. *Second:* Write a number 1 in front of item numbers not circled if you responded A (always) or F (frequently). Circle the number 1's which you have written in front of the following items: 3, 5, 8, 10, 15, 18, 19, 22, 24, 26, 28, 30, 32, 34, and 35. *Third:* Count the circled number 1's. This is your score for concern for people. Record the score in the blank following the letter P at the end of the questionnaire. *Fourth:* Count the uncircled number 1's. This is your score for concern for task. Record this number in the blank following the letter T.

Awareness of your leadership style will help you to tailor your responses in personal or work situations. You will be able to compare your perception of how people and task oriented you are with a score of how you respond in specific situations. The next step is to determine if your score matches your desired response and determine whether to continue your present leadership style or to make changes to become more participate (if you score high on autocratic leadership style) or more directive (if you score high on laissez-faire leadership style).

Task Orientation and People Orientation Leadership-Style Profile Sheet

Directions: To determine your style of leadership, mark your score on the concern for task dimension (T) on the left-hand arrow below. Next, move to the right-hand arrow and mark your score on the concern for people dimension (P). Draw a straight line that intersects the P and T scores. The point at which that line crosses the shared leadership arrow indicates your score on that dimension.

Shared Leadership Results From Balancing Concern for Task and Concern for People

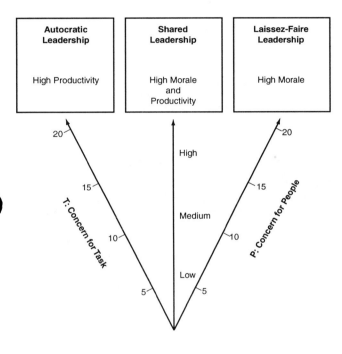

CASE STUDY

Jennifer is the nurse manager of a 68-bed respiratory unit who has responsibility for 95 employees. Jennifer tailors her leadership style according to the employees' needs, experience, and situation. She is helping a graduate nurse who is on orientation to learn how to use the documentation forms. Jennifer provides detailed instructions to the new nurse, explaining step-by-step the process for documentation. In another situation, Jennifer asks a seasoned clinical nurse to take responsibility for the total quality improvement process. She provides the nurse with information and offers to assist anytime the clinical nurse needs consultation. Jennifer promotes Susan, a clinical nurse, to a 3-11 charge position. Since this is Susan's first management experience, Jennifer is providing a structured orientation, but is giving Susan the opportunity to seek out the information Susan needs and to design learning objectives to meet Susan's needs.

Situational leadership
Democratic
Authoritative

Case Study Questions

1. What type of leadership theory is Jennifer using?
2. What are the benefits of changing the leadership style based on the employee's experience, knowledge, and situation? *more effective rather than one-style.*

LEARNING RESOURCES

Discussion Questions

1. Is a clinical nurse a leader?
2. What are the characteristics of effective leaders? Identify an effective leader.
3. What is situational leadership? Are the three styles of leadership—authoritarian, democratic, and laissez-faire—interchangeable? What are the differences?
4. How can nursing as a profession exhibit leadership in defining policy for healthcare delivery?
5. According to Kouzes & Posner, what are the five practices common to exceptional leadership achievements?
   risk taking
   empowering
   visions
   change
   motivating groups

Reproduced from *A Handbook of Structured Experiences for Human Relations Training,* vol. 1, by J.W. Pfeiffer & J.E. Jones (eds.). Copyright © 1974 by Pfeiffer & Company, San Diego, CA. The T-P Leadership Questionnaire was adapted from Sergiovanni, Metzcus, and Burden's revision of the Leadership Behavior Description Questionnaire, *American Educational Research Journal* 6 (1969), pages 62–79.

Study Questions

Fill in the Blank: Identify the appropriate leadership style for the following situations.

1. A code has been called. Which leadership style is most effective in this situation? _____

   autocratic (direct leadership)

2. The nursing record is being revised. Which leadership style is most appropriate? _____

   democratic (direction is needed through facilitation & coordination

3. Nurses, physicians, dietitians, and social workers are working together to increase patient services in a hospital. Which leadership style is useful? *democratic or laissez-faire to provide direction, but allow group leadership & team work*

True and False: Circle the correct answer.

T̄ F 1. Two critical skills in leadership are interpersonal and problem-solving skills.

T (F) 2. Followership is a process whereby leaders participate in group decisions.

T (F) 3. Empowerment is the ability to lead a group successfully.

(T) F 4. Important skills for leading include diagnosing, adapting, and communicating.

(T) F 5. Situational leaders tailor their leadership style based upon the employee, experience, and situation.

T (F) 6. Laissez-faire leadership entails minimal participation and directing by the leader resulting in high productivity.

T (F) 7. A transactional leader is one who motivates employees to their full potential.

SUPPLEMENTAL READINGS

Corser, W.D. (1995). First-Line managers: What do nurses expect?, *Nursing Management, 25*(3), 32-36.

Kison, C. (1980). Leadership: How, who and what? *Nursing Management, 20*(11), 72-74.

Kouzes, J. & Posner, B. (1988). *The leadership practices inventory.* San Diego, CA: Pfeiffer & Company.

Chapter 5

Management Principles

STUDY FOCUS

Management is the coordination and integration of resources through planning, organizing, directing, and controlling in order to accomplish specific organizational goals and objectives. Nursing management is coordinating and integrating nursing resources by applying the management process to organize and deliver high quality client care to individuals, groups, and communities. The management process is composed of four steps: planning, organizing, directing, and controlling. A major task of management is to link the staff at the bottom of the organization with those at the top. Nurse managers must continuously balance two important, and at times competing, needs: those of the staff for growth and those of the organization for viability.

Planning for the needs of individuals and the organization is complex and requires time and skill. Strategic planning is a long-term process which provides direction and purpose for the organization. Tactical planning is typically a short-term process and focuses on the specific details of activities necessary to accomplish the broad organizational goals. In order to accomplish goals, the manager must organize the integration and coordination of resources. Organization is the mobilization of the human, financial, and material resources of the agency to achieve established goals. Directing employees by motivating and providing leadership is essential to goal accomplishment. Nurse managers must know the scope of nursing practice to assign and delegate tasks to appropriate personnel. After the nurse manager has assigned work to staff, and goals have been accomplished, evaluation of the outcomes is necessary. Controlling refers to examining the results of activities (outcomes) in light of a predetermined standard for the purpose of quality control and then taking corrective actions when necessary.

A nurse manager is a registered nurse who holds 24-hour accountability for management of a healthcare unit(s). The nurse manager's role is complex and varied encompassing multiple diverse tasks, many of which require immediate action. The components of the nurse manager role include managing care delivery; managing resources; developing personnel; complying with regulatory and professional standards; and fostering interdisciplinary and collaborative relationships. Mintzberg (1975) identifies ten important role behaviors for managers which he categorizes into three role sets. The role sets are: interpersonal (figurehead, leader, and liaison), informational (monitor, disseminator, and spokesperson), and decisional (entrepreneur, disturbance handler, resource allocator, and negotiator).

Managing difficult individuals is a challenging task for any manager. Difficult individuals may exhibit negative attitudes or behaviors. Lewis-Ford (1993) describes the following categories of difficult people: Sherman tanks, snipers, exploders, bulldozers, balloons, clams, negative nabobs, complainers, and stallers. Tactics to use with these individuals include trying to understand their behavior, preparing yourself psychologically to interact with them, and selecting disciplinary measures, if necessary.

Time management is an extremely important part of a manager's position. Managers who do not manage their own time end up being controlled by circumstances, situations, and crises. Major timesavers include setting goals, prioritizing activities, and planning. Major time robbers include wasted effort, unproductive meetings, crisis orientation, and interruptions. Effectively planning, prioritizing, and scheduling time is essential for individuals who want to accomplish personal and professional goals.

LEARNING TOOLS

Self-assessment

Managing Time

Introduction: Organizing one's time is extremely crucial. Time is a valuable asset. In the Western culture, we believe that time comes and goes; once it is gone, we cannot recover the moment. For individuals to effectively manage time, they must first determine what personal and professional goals are important for them to accomplish. This self-assessment includes three parts: identifying and prioritizing personal and professional goals; logging activities and amounts of time for each; and identifying and prioritizing activities.

Part I

Directions: Complete the following task: In the blank lines below, identify and prioritize by ranking five personal and professional goals for three time periods.

1 Year Personal Goals	5 Year Personal Goals	Lifetime Personal Goals
1.	1.	1.
2.	2.	2.
3.	3.	3.
4.	4.	4.
5.	5.	5.

1 Year Professional Goals	5 Year Professional Goals	Lifetime Professional Goals
1.	1.	1.
2.	2.	2.
3.	3.	3.
4.	4.	4.
5.	5.	5.

The task of identifying and prioritizing your personal and professional goals is very time consuming and difficult, but essential for you to manage your time effectively. Annually you should revisit your list and update as well as congratulate yourself on accomplishments.

Part II

Directions: For a 24-hour period write down all activities that you complete as well as the time you engaged in the activity in a small notebook. After you have made a 24-hour record, determine the number of minutes engaged in each activity. A sample log is illustrated below.

Time Started	Time Completed	Activity	Total Time in Minutes

This activity is useful in at least three ways. First, it identifies any time robbers such as interruptions, unproductive meetings, telephone solicitations, unorganized activities, and time wasters that may be filling your day. Secondly, it shows you what activities you chose to spend your time doing. That way you can compare these activities to your personal and professional goals to see if they are congruent, or if you need to reprioritize your activities. Finally, it shows you your style of time management. Are you managing a crisis constantly? Are you spending all of your time in professional activities? How much personal time do you have?

Part III

Directions: Identify those personal and professional activities that are most important to you and prioritize them. This is the easy task because you have already established your goals. Now, make a daily or weekly list of activities that you need to accomplish and check them off as they are completed. This check list should be a tool and should not become the center of time management. Below is an example of a check list. You may rank your activities according to their priority or star those that are most critical to complete first.

This activity helps to organize your daily and weekly workload into a manageable list.

Activities to Accomplish	Date to be Completed	Check when Completed
1. _____	_____	_____
2. _____	_____	_____
3. _____	_____	_____
4. _____	_____	_____
5. _____	_____	_____
6. _____	_____	_____
7. _____	_____	_____
8. _____	_____	_____
9. _____	_____	_____
10. _____	_____	_____

CASE STUDY

Ruth Anne is a nurse manager of an oncology unit for Middle View Hospital in North Dakota. Ruth Anne has been a manager for fifteen years and enjoys the role. She is proud of the fact that she has never once been over budget at year end, has maintained a high productivity level, and has a stable core staff. Ruth Anne is very detail-oriented and organized. Ruth Anne conscientiously follows policies and procedures, and implements new programs according to protocol. She meets monthly with the director of the medical surgical areas and keeps her abreast of any changes in the unit. Ruth Anne is open to new trial innovations that the director asks her to initiate. Ruth Anne treats all employees equitably and follows the personnel handbook for any human resource issue.

Case Study Questions

1. Does Ruth Anne exhibit managerial or leadership behaviors?
2. What management behaviors does she exhibit?

LEARNING RESOURCES

Discussion Questions

1. What are effective ways to manage your time? What are examples of time robbers? Why is it important to manage your time effectively?
2. What are some categories of difficult people? What are some effective methods to manage difficult people?
3. What is the management process? What is involved in each of the four steps?

4. What is the role of a nurse manager? What is the nature of managerial work?
5. How do management and leadership differ? Are there similarities between leadership and management?

Study Questions

True and False: Circle the correct answer.

T ~~F~~ 1. Leadership is more important than management in a turbulent health-care environment.

T ~~F~~ 2. Transformational leaders focus on themaintenance of quality and quantity of performance.

~~T~~ F 3. Transformational leadership is necessary in periods of growth, change, and crisis.

~~T~~ F 4. Management is focused on tasks and accomplishing organizational goals.

T ~~F~~ 5. Nursing management is the coordination and integration of resources using a political and computer science process.

~~T~~ F 6. The traditional management functions include planning, organizing, controlling, and coordinating.

T ~~F~~ 7. Tactical planning is a broad-range process of establishing the purpose and direction of the organization.

~~T~~ F 8. Time management requires the disciplined use of time and the scheduling of priority activities.

T ~~F~~ 9. Causes of time mismanagement include setting goals, unproductive meetings, and crisis orientation.

~~T~~ F 10. Nurse managers usually have 24-hour accountability for the coordination and delivery of care.

SUPPLEMENTAL READINGS

Dienemann, J. (1992). Manager responsibilities in community agencies and hospitals. *Journal of Nursing Administration*, 22(5), 40-45.

Lewis-Ford, B. (1993). Management techniques: Coping with difficult people. *Nursing Management*, 24(3), 36-38.

Mintzberg, H. (1975). The manager's job: Folklore and fact. In M. Matteson and J. Ivancevich (Eds.), *Management classics* (3rd ed.) (pp. 63-85). Plano, TX: Business Publications.

Tumulty, G. (1992). Head nurse role redesign: Improving satisfaction and performance. *Journal of Nursing Administration*, 22(2), 41-65.

Chapter 6

Problem Solving

STUDY FOCUS

A problem is a deficit or surplus of something that is needed to achieve one's goals. We encounter problems daily in our personal and professional lives. Some situations produce problems (a difficulty), some problems create conflict (a dilemma), and sometimes an individual's solution does not take a logical path (a paradox). Solving problems effectively is important to making good client care decisions. Solving problems is a rational-logical thought process. There are six steps in the problem-solving process. The first step is to gather information from a variety of sources and to analyze that data. The second step is to define the problem by clarifying the task and describing it in a single sentence. Thirdly, develop potential solutions in order to make the single best choice. The fourth step is to consider the consequences for each of the identified potential solutions. Making the single best decision is the fifth step. Finally, implement the solution, evaluate its effectiveness, and take necessary corrective action.

The Kirton Adaptation-Innovation Theory identifies two types of problem-solving styles, adapting and innovating. Adaptors use more traditional approaches to problem solving. They do not seek out problems to solve, but do resolve the problems they confront. In contrast, innovators seek novel situations, challenge rules, and create solutions. They discover problems and attack them vigorously. Problem solvers typically assess problems by their urgency and their immediacy. Some people envision problems on a time continuum. On one end of the continuum is a potential problem which may emerge at any time; in the middle are actual problems that require prompt attention; and on the far end are critical problems which are extremely urgent and require crisis intervention.

There are many strategies that can be used to solve problems. Some of the most common problem-solving strategies include direct intervention, indirect intervention, delegation, purposeful inaction, and consultation or collaboration. Direct intervention involves you personally doing a task or activity. Indirect intervention requires good interpersonal skills — negotia-

tion, conflict resolution, persuasion, and confrontation — to influence others to carry out activities or resolve the problem. Delegation is used to assign the responsibility of an activity or task to another for the purpose of workload distribution. Purposeful inaction is consciously ignoring or choosing not to make a choice with the hope that the problem may go away with time. Inaction can be useful in some situations. Consultation or collaboration is exchanging information with peers and colleagues in order to solve a problem.

In today's healthcare environment, team-based approaches to patient care are commonplace. Nurses must learn to function and solve problems effectively in group environments. Dailey (1990) describes a nine-step problem-solving procedure to solve problems in group/team settings. The steps include: 1) identifying problems, 2) determining perceptions, 3) determining the underlying causes of problems, 4) assessing the magnitude of the problem, 5) constructing a plan, 6) implementing a plan, 7) test piloting the plan after discussing it with the team, 8) tracking effectiveness by creating indicators, and 9) publicizing results.

LEARNING TOOLS

Self-assessment

Problem-Solving In-Basket Exercise

Introduction: Nurses are confronted daily with multiple problems, not only in their personal lives, but in their professional work as well. Diagnostic reasoning and clinical decision making are skills needed by all registered nurses. In-basket exercises are useful for improving skills.

1. Read the memos below, and then identify which problem type they are — potential, actual, or critical.

2. Take the critical problem you identify, and use the six-step problem-solving process to work it through. This exercise will give you practice in identifying types of problems and skill in solving them.

You arrive on the unit, check your mail, and find the following memos:

Memo 1
From: Nancy, Head Nurse of 4 West
To: Sue, Staff Nurse
Re: Quality Improvement
   Sue, as the 4 West representative to the hospital's quality improvement team, one of your responsibilities is to monitor documentation on the nursing flow chart, and alert and assist nurses to comply with our unit standards. In the most recent report, I noticed that 4 West has a poor rate of compliance. Please attend to this situation immediately. **(What type of problem is this? _____)**

Memo 2
From: Jon, Personnel Director
To: Sue, Staff Nurse–4 West
Re: Health Insurance
   Sue, it has come to my attention that two of your health insurance enrollment forms were incorrectly completed. We have submitted the required data, and you have insurance coverage, but the records should be completed properly sometime in the future. **(What type of problem is this? _____)**

Verbal Report 3
   Sylvia stops you in the hall and tells you that Mrs. N's family is displeased with her care. They are demanding to speak to someone in charge. Sylvia is in a hurry to get home because she has a sick child and quickly leaves. **(What type of problem is this? _____)**

   Directions: Determine the most critical of the three problems identified above. Write the name of the problem below. Then use the six-step problem-solving process to resolve it.

Problem-solving Steps

Decision Name:

1. Gather information. _____
   _____

2. Define problem. _____
   _____

3. Develop solutions. _____
   _____

4. Consider consequences. _____
   _____

5. Make a decision. _____
   _____

6. Implement and evaluate solution. _____
   _____

CASE STUDY

   Beth is a nurse manager for the cardiac intensive care unit in a large teaching hospital in Birmingham, Alabama. She enjoys challenges, pushes her staff to maximum productivity, and works at least ten-hour shifts. If the organizational rules are in her way, she challenges them and works toward an innovative solution to the problem. Beth enjoys novel situations rather than routine or day-to-day challenges. She seems to thrive on unique problems and designs creative solutions to solve them. The staff on the cardiac intensive care unit like Beth's style and support her in her efforts.

Case Study Questions

1. According to Kirton's Adaptation-Innovation Theory, what type of problem-solving style is Beth exhibiting?
2. Describe the similarities and differences of adaptors and innovators.

LEARNING RESOURCES

Discussion Questions

1. In what situations would a nurse use the problem-solving process as opposed to the team problem-solving process?
2. How do the steps of the problem-solving process, the nursing process, and the team problem-solving process differ? How are they similar?
3. What are some strategies that can be used to solve problems? Give examples of a situation in which these strategies would be useful.
4. Is it important for nurses to have diagnostic reasoning and clinical decision-making skills? If yes, why?
5. Should nurses consider the economic implications when providing client care?

Study Questions

Matching: Write the letter of the correct response in front of each term.

G 1. Problem Solving
C 2. Actual Problem
E 3. Adaptor
F 4. Innovator
D 5. Delegation
B 6. Potential Problem
A 7. Critical Problem

A. a situation that is highly urgent and needs crisis intervention

B. a situation that is tenuous and difficulties can occur at any time

C. a situation that occurs in real time and needs prompt action

D. assigning responsibilities and tasks to others

E. uses tried and accepted solutions to problems

F. uses innovative, creative solutions to problems

G. using a process to identify obstacles and to achieve goals

True and False: Circle the correct answer.

 T   F   1. Problem solving is a rational-logical thought process.

T   F   2. It is inappropriate for a manager to use indirect intervention to solve problems.

T   F   3. Purposeful inaction is an extremely valuable tool in most situations.

SUPPLEMENTAL READINGS

Dailey, R. (1990). Strengthening hospital nursing: How to use problem-solving teams effectively. *Journal of Nursing Administration, 20*(7/8), 24-29.

Kirton, M. (1989). *Adaptors and innovators: Styles of creativity and problem solving.* London: Routledge.

Marquis, B.L. & Huston, C.L. (Summer, 1994). Decisions, decisions, decisions. *Advance Practice Nurse,* 46-49.

Chapter 7

Decision Making

STUDY FOCUS

Decision making is selecting from among competing alternative solutions and then implementing activities to accomplish your goal. Decision making not only deals with problems, but opportunities, challenges, and leadership initiatives as well. Decision making has five core elements: identifying a problem, establishing criteria to evaluate potential solutions, searching for alternative solutions, evaluating alternatives, and selecting the single best choice. Individuals frame problems in different ways. One way is to use a systems approach like those used in quality improvement processes where emphasis is placed on the organizational process and groups problem solving. Another method of framing a problem is to view the decision as individual rather than organizational. In an individual problem, all responsibility, accountability, and decision-making authority rests with one person.

According to Wren (1974), there are ten steps in the decision-making process: 1) becoming aware of a situation, 2) investigating the nature of the situation, 3) determining the objectives of the solution, 4) determining alternative solutions, 5) weighing the consequences and relative efficiency of each solution, 6) evaluating various alternatives, 7) selecting the best alternative, 8) implementing the decision, 9) evaluating the solution, and 10) correcting the solution based on evaluation. Nurses use the decision-making process for individual, clinical, and organizational problem solving. Clinical decision making or clinical judgment is decision making based on nurse and client interaction and goal setting. Some nurses use diagnostic reasoning in their practice. Diagnostic reasoning is a four-step process that includes attending to available cues, activating hypotheses, gathering data, and evaluating hypotheses with data until a diagnosis is reached (Elstein, Shulman & Sprafka, 1978). Organizational decision making is assessing and solving systems problems to attain agency goals. Ethical decision making is examining conflicts among ethical principles, resource allocation decisions, and values.

Administrative decision making is commonly made under conditions of uncertainty, has high risk, and involves the allocation of human, financial, and/or material resources. Four types of administrative decision-making strategies include satisficing, incrementalism, mixed scanning, and optimizing. Satisficing is getting by, selecting a solution that is good enough. Incrementalism is a slow step-by-step approach to solving an immediate problem with progress toward an optimal course of action. Mixed scanning combines an opportunistic approach to problem solving with the goal of optimizing the results. Optimizing entails choosing the course of action with the highest payoff.

One may engage in many different strategies when making decisions. Formal decision strategies include trial and error, pilot projects, problem critique, creativity techniques, the decision tree, the fish bone or cause-and-effect chart, group decision making, cost-benefit analysis, and worst-case scenarios. Trial-and-error strategies involve selecting the first available solution and trying it on the problem. Many times this approach results in poor outcomes. Pilot projects are minirepresentations of a formal project. One unit is selected to implement the project thereby minimizing risk and providing an opportunity to identify problems. Problem critique is a technique where a decision maker describes a potential solution for the problem to a friend or colleague, and then they critique the solution. Multiple creativity techniques include nominal group, Delphi, and brainstorming. The goal of creativity techniques is to identify as many potential solutions as possible without threatening individuals or critiquing responses. A decision tree is a graphic model of a problem's options, outcomes, and risks. Critical paths are examples of decision trees. Fish bone or cause-and-effect charts are graphic figures diagrammed as a sentence is with horizontal and slanted lines. The diagram represents the product, process, and outcome. Fish bones are used to diagnose causes of production problems. Group decision making is a process that engages the group to take ownership for organizational problems. Cost-benefit analysis is the process of identifying the costs and benefits of a solution to determine the fiscal, human, and material impact. Driving and restraining forces are also identified. Worst-case scenarios are typically used when money or prestige is at stake. Decision makers examine all possible events that could go wrong in order to determine a course of action that will protect the organization.

Nurses may also use the tools of perception and innovation in their decision making. These tools enable nurses to break out of their traditional decision-making strategies by finding novel solutions that provide a high payoff. Perception affects how one views the solution. Reframing one's perception of the problem or solution can create a new method to solve problems and may lead to the creation of a new device or new business. Innovations are those activities that have not been tried before in the same form. Reframing problems and solutions is a key strategy to change the way we perceive and select solutions.

LEARNING TOOLS

Group Activity: Understanding Decision Making

Purpose: To identify the different types of decisions and to determine which decision situations are more appropriate for individual and group decision making.

Directions: For the three decision situations described below, identify the type of decision (administrative, clinical, or ethical), and who is the appropriate decision maker (individual or group).

Decision 1

Mr. Smith is in a nursing home. He is 72 years old and had a cerebral vascular accident three months ago which left him comatose. Mr. Smith has a feeding tube, and tube feedings are given on a regular basis. Mrs. Smith visited today and stated that she does not want you to give him tube feedings anymore because he wouldn't want to live "like this." What should you do?

Type of Decision _____

Decision Maker _____

Decision 2

Mr. Jones returned from surgery eight hours ago. He had a left total knee replacement and now is complaining of excruciating pain. He is requesting pain medication. What should you do?

Type of Decision _____

Decision Maker _____

Decision 3

You are the team leader on an orthopedic unit for the 3-11 shift. All the nurses have been complaining of being overworked. At 11:35 P.M., all the nurses are gathered at the exit waiting for you. They are upset and demand that something be done about the chronic short staffing. What should you do?

Type of Decision _____

Decision Maker _____

As a nurse, you will be confronted with the need to make many different decisions. Determining quickly which decisions you can act upon by yourself and determining which ones need to be handled by a group is crucial to your success.

CASE STUDY

Dawn is a nurse manager for the operating room of a small community hospital in Oshkosh, Wisconsin. Dawn is required to make many administrative decisions daily. Dawn prefers to make administrative decisions by using a step-by-step approach to solving immediate problems, using solutions that fit into her long-range goals. For example, staffing problems have arisen in the operating room. Dawn's long-range goal is to have a mix of operating room technicians and registered nurses in the operating room to provide quality perioperative care. Today, Dawn will begin discussing her plans with the staff, but in the meantime, will cover the staffing need with an experienced registered nurse from intensive care to assist in covering the holding room area. Dawn's experience suggests that taking small steps to solve a problem is useful and gives her an opportunity to reflect on opportunities and barriers.

Case Study Questions

1. In administrative decision making, there are four strategies commonly used to make decisions. Which is Dawn using?
2. Describe the other administrative decision making strategies.

LEARNING RESOURCES

Discussion Questions

1. How can you use the tools of perception and innovation in your nursing practice?
2. What is the difference between an individual and organizational problem? Give an example of each.
3. Describe the formal strategies of decision making, and provide an example of a situation in which each would be useful.
4. Discuss the problem-solving and decision-making processes. Are there similarities? Differences?
5. What types of decisions should clinical nurses make? Who should a clinical nurse turn to for assistance in decision making?

Study Questions

True and False: Circle the correct answer.

T (F) 1. Clinical decision making is the same thing as diagnostic reasoning.

(T) F 2. Organizational decision making focuses on system problems.

(T) F 3. Ethical decision making is influenced by each person's values.

T (F) 4. Administrative decision making focuses on clinical problems.

(T) F 5. Critical pathways are a form of decision tree.

(T) F 6. Group decision making tends to be more effective for system problems.

T (F) 7. In most cases, satisficing leads to effective decision making.

T (F) 8. Administrative decisions tend to be clear cut and easy to solve.

T (F) 9. Decision-making strategies are interchangeable and can be used effectively in any situation.

T (F) 10. Pilot projects are full scale implementations of a solution.

SUPPLEMENTAL READINGS

Jacobs, S. & Pelfrey, S. (1995). Decision support systems: Using computers to help manage. *Journal of Nursing Administration, 25(2)*, 46-51.

Janis, I. & Mann, L. (1977) *Decision making: A psychological analysis of conflict, choice, and commitment.* New York: Free Press.

Showemaker, P. & Russo, J. (1993). A pyramid of decision approaches. *California Management Review, 36(1)*, 9-31.

Wren, G. (1974). *Modern health administration.* Athens, GA: University of Georgia Press.

Chapter 8

The Use of Groups, Committees, and Teams

STUDY FOCUS

Healthcare delivery systems are becoming more complex, requiring multidisciplinary work teams to tackle difficult systems problems in a cost-controlled manner. In most healthcare environments, nursing is at the core of client care, providing around-the-clock access to healthcare services. As central players in the delivery of client care, nurses are expected to assume the role of team leaders, case managers, and coordinators of care. Many of the care-coordinating roles entail interdisciplinary consultation and intense group work.

A group is a collection of interrelated individuals working toward a goal. Group interactions are composed of five elements: process, standards, decision making, communication, and roles (Book & Galvin, 1975). Process is the way the group works together to accomplish goals. Standards are values and norms that the group uses to process information. Decision making is the method the group uses to solve problems. Communication includes verbal and non-verbal interactions, both within and external to the group. Roles describe each individual's part in the group. Creative techniques used by groups to enhance group process and improve outcomes include brainstorming, nominal group technique, tri-council, and the delphi survey.

Groups progress through a series of four stages: orientation, adaptation, emergence, and working (Farley & Stoner, 1989). The orientation stage occurs at the beginning of the group's formation and involves trust and boundary issues. During adaptation, a team's identity is formed and individual roles are differentiated. In the emergence control phase, issues arise and are resolved. The working phase is the productive stage when decision making and task accomplishment take place. These stages of the group process are not necessarily sequential and may be iterative.

People join groups for a variety of reasons. Oftentimes people seek group participation to fulfill affilia-

tion and achievement needs. When individuals work in groups, they gain the advantage of a greater depth and breadth of knowledge and information. Also, members of groups tend to accept and endorse group solutions to problems because of their commitment and investment in the decision-making process. Complex problems are more manageable within groups because they tend to have an increased knowledge base and a varied approach to problem solving. In groups, individuals are provided with the outlet for an expression of ideas. The disadvantages of groups can include premature decision making, individual domination and control, and disruptive conflicts. Individuals will belong to groups as long as their needs are being met. Once the costs of membership become greater than the benefits, termination will likely occur.

Much of group work is organized and completed through meetings. Meetings are typically held to disseminate information, seek opinions, and solve problems. The important components of a successful meeting are distribution of an agenda, careful selection of members, attention to starting times and seating positions, and facilitation of discussion of the issues. Committees are formally designated groups. Committees meet at scheduled times and have an identified purpose. Task forces or ad hoc committees are specially formed to respond to a pressing need. Once the need is met, the task force is disbanded.

A continuum of authority in group decision making includes the autocratic, the consultative, the joint, and the delegated styles. The leader's style of facilitating the group's decision making affects the power of the group. The leader's role is pivotal in facilitating positive work groups to accomplish organizational goals. The leader must redirect disruptive group members such as compulsive talkers, nontalkers, interrupters, squashers, and busybodies. Team building is an essential component of the group leader's role.

LEARNING TOOLS

Group Activity: Winter Survival Decision Exercise

Purpose: To compare autocratic, consultative, joint, and delegated group decision making authority.

1. Divide the study group into four small groups of seven to twelve. One member of each small group will be the designated leader; one member will be the designated observer; and all other members will be participants in the small group during this exercise. Group 1 should be assigned autocratic group decision authority; Group 2 should be assigned consultative group decision authority; Group 3 should be assigned joint group decision authority; and Group 4 should be assigned delegated group decision-making authority.

2. The observer should be attuned to the process by which the groups make decisions. Crucial issues are how well the group uses the resources of its members, how much commitment to implement the decision is mustered, how the future decision-making ability of the group is affected, and how members feel about and react to what is taking place. The observer should address the following issues: Who does and does not participate in discussion? Who participates most? Who participates least? Who influences the decision? Who does not influence the decision? How is influence determined (expertise, loudness)? What are the dominant group feelings? What resources are used to make a decision?

3. Give each group the following exercise and the Winter Survival Decision Form:

You have crash-landed into a lake in the northern Minnesota and southern Manitoba woods. It is ll:32 A.M. in mid-January. The light plane in which you were traveling crashed on a lake. The pilot and copilot of the light plane were killed. Shortly after the crash, the plane sinks completely into the lake with the pilot's and copilot's bodies inside. None of you are seriously injured, and you are all dry.

The crash came suddenly, before the pilot had time to radio for help or inform anyone of your position. Since your pilot was trying to avoid a storm, you know the plane was considerably off course. The pilot announced shortly before the crash that you were twenty miles northwest of a small town that is the nearest known habitation.

You are in a wilderness area made up of thick woods broken by many lakes and streams. The snow depth varies from above the ankles in windswept areas to knee-deep where it has drifted. The last weather report indicated that the temperature would reach –25°F in the daytime and –40° at night. Plenty of dead wood and twigs are in the immediate area. You are dressed in winter clothing appropriate for city wear — suits, pantsuits, street shoes, and overcoats.

While escaping from the plane, several members of your group salvaged twelve items. Your task is to rank these items according to their importance to your survival. You may assume that the number of passengers is the same as the number of persons in your group and that the group has agreed to stick together.

Winter Survival Decision Form

Directions: Rank the following items according to their importance to your survival, starting with 1 for the most important item and proceeding to 12 for the least important item.

____ Ball of steel wool

____ Newspapers (one per person)

____ Compass

____ Hand ax

____ Cigarette lighter (without fluid)

____ Loaded .45 caliber pistol

____ Sectional air map made of plastic

____ Twenty-by-twenty-foot piece of heavy-duty canvas

____ Extra shirts and pants for each survivor

____ Can of shortening

____ Quart of l00-proof whiskey

____ Family-size chocolate bars (one per person)

4. Provide 45 minutes for each group to work through this exercise, then ask them to score their answers.

Scoring: Score the net difference between the participants' answers and the correct answer. For example, if a participant's answer is 9 and the correct answer is 12, the net difference is 3. Disregard all plus or minus signs. Find only the net difference for each item. Total all the item scores. The lower the score the more accurate the ranking.

Winter Survival Exercise: Answer Key

Item	Expert Ranking	Your Rank	Difference Score
Ball of steel wool	2		
Newspaper (one per person)	8		
Compass	12		
Hand ax	6		
Cigarette lighter (without fluid)	1		
Loaded .45-caliber pistol	9		
Sectional air map made of plastic	11		
Twenty-by-twenty foot piece of heavy-duty canvas	5		
Extra shirt and pants for each survivor	3		
Can of shortening	4		
Quart of 100-proof whiskey	10		
Family-size chocolate bar (one per person)	7		
Total			

5. Have the observer brief the small groups with his or her observations. This is a good time to discuss effective group decision-making techniques. Provide 15 minutes for this activity.

6. Get the total group back together, and have the leader of each group share their group scores, the type of group decision-making authority that their group were role-playing, and key observations made by the observers of their small groups.

(From Johnson, D.W. & Johnson, F.P. *Joining Together: Group Theory and Group Skills*, third edition. Copyright © 1986. All rights reserved. Adapted by permission of Allyn & Bacon.)

CASE STUDY

Jackie, a Nurse Practitioner who works in a primary care setting, feels isolated from other Nurse Practitioners because there are only physician assistants and physicians where she is employed. Jackie organizes a Nurse Practitioner group, invites other Nurse Practitioners to attend, and arranges the meeting place. The first meeting is a formal organizational gathering where people introduce themselves, socialize, and become familiar with one another and the purpose for the group. Goals are set and roles are assigned at the second, third, and fourth meetings. During the next several meetings, a number of individuals try to control the issues that are to be addressed. Once the issues are determined and people agree to be responsible for tasks, the work progresses quickly, and the group feels a sense of accomplishment.

Case Study Questions

1. What stages did this group work through?
2. What are the four stages of group progress, and what do they include?
3. Do groups progress sequentially through the stages?

LEARNING RESOURCES

Discussion Questions

1. What is the continuum of authority for group decision making? How does the leader's style of facilitating the group affect group decision-making authority?
2. What are the types of disruptive group members, and what are strategies to redirect their energy toward group work and goal accomplishment?
3. What are the possible roles for clinical nurses in an interdisciplinary team?
4. What is the difference between a meeting, a committee, and a task force?
5. What are the stages of group development? Provide leader strategies to facilitate the group process for each stage.
6. What are the advantages and disadvantages of group work?
7. Describe the leader's role in planning and conducting a meeting.

Study Questions

True or False: Circle the correct answer.

(T) F   1. Interdisciplinary work teams are necessary for complex situations.

T (F)   2. Groups sequentially go through the stages of orientation, adaptation, emergence, and working.

T (F)   3. The major reason people join groups is to gain information.

T (F)   4. Group decision making is cost effective in all situations.

(T) F   5. A group leader must organize and structure a group for success.

T (F)   6. In all groups, decision making is a joint process with all members participating.

(T) F   7. A committee is a formally designated group designed to meet organizational objectives.

T (F)   8. A task force is designed to solve long-term problems.

(T) F   9. Team building is a complex process that requires leader and group commitment and cooperation.

T (F) 10. The ideal number of members in a group is between 10–14.

SUPPLEMENTAL READINGS

Book, C. & Galvin, K. (1975). *Instruction in and about small group discussion.* Falls Church, VA: Speech Communication Association.

Farley, M. & Stoner, M. (1989). The nurse executive and interdisciplinary team building. *Nursing Administration Quarterly, 13*(2), 24-30.

Gaynor, S.E., Reschak, G.L., & Verdin, J. (1994). Evaluating a committee structure. *Journal of Nursing Administration, 24*(7/8), 59-63.

Johnson, D.W. & Johnson, F.P. (1987). *Joining Together.* New Jersey: Prentice-Hall, Inc.

Chapter 9

Budgeting and Financial Management

STUDY FOCUS

Budgeting and financial management are crucial skills for nurses who practice the art and science of nursing. In healthcare, resources are scarce; reimbursement structures have changed; and organizations are seeking methods to cut costs. How then can a nurse manager justify expenses, garner new resources, and compete with other healthcare managers for limited dollars? A strong foundation in financial management is essential.

Financial management is a set of activities involving the allocation of resources to complete organizational objectives and ensure viability. Four phases of financial management are budgeting, recording, reporting, and evaluating. To maximize the use of limited resources, organizations engage in planning. Operational plans are those activities determined necessary for meeting day-to-day organizational goals. Strategic planning is more long-term and entails analyzing and projecting future organizational goals. A budget puts planning into financial terms and provides direction for managers. A budget is a written plan of revenues and expenditures. Expenses are those costs incurred to meet organizational goals. Revenues are payments made by patients and insurance companies for services rendered or amounts still owed for a service that was provided. Profits exist when revenues exceed costs of labor, material, and overhead expenses.

There are three types of budgets: cash, capital and expense. A cash budget logs cash receipts and disbursements. A capital budget involves the purchase of big ticket items like buildings, land, or large costly pieces of equipment. In many organizations, a capital purchase is any item greater than $500. The expense budget is a record of expenditures for human or material resources. Managers also track direct and indirect expenses. Direct costs are those items that result in providing physical care to the client. Indirect costs include overhead, supportive, and administrative expenses. Nurse managers also measure the intensity of care by examining the amount, type, and cost of nursing care for client groups.

Some of the largest expenditures in healthcare organization budgets are controlled by nurses who oversee nursing personnel and supply usage. The large size of nursing departments puts nurses at risk for lay-offs and downsizing. Nurses will be called upon to contain costs and provide high quality healthcare. Suggestions for nurses that promote cost control include doing a job efficiently, motivating clients to recover, using supplies carefully, and maximizing the use of time. Nurse managers may also cost out nursing services to determine the actual "cost" of care provided by client type.

Familiarity with the three basic types of budgets will assist nurse managers when interacting with financial personnel. Traditional budgets are based on expenses for the previous year with an inflation factor added. Zero-based budgets require the manager to rebuild the budget each year justifying all line items. Performance budgets are based on the activities of a cost center. The budgetary process involves four phases: disseminating instructions, preparing the first budget draft, reviewing and adjusting, and appealing. There are two key components of budgeting — volume and cost measures. Volume measures are activity standards based on a workload measure for the organization. The cost measure is commonly a salary standard.

LEARNING TOOLS

Reporting Exercise

Purpose: To identify the important categories of a monthly manager's report and to identify important data for each category.

Introduction: Nurse managers have 24-hour accountability for the staffing, management, and leadership of their assigned unit(s). They are to be fiscally responsible and must manage their resources to stay within budget or within the adjusted budget based on client days, adjustments in acuity, and length of stay. Most managers are held accountable in four major categories: financial, material, human, and unit goals. The financial data category reflects the actual versus budgeted expenses for each line item (such as equipment, supplies, salaries). Variances both positive and negative are reported and justified. The material data category reports changes in products or supplies, any equipment trials or examinations, and any changes in procedures for the unit(s). The human resource category reflects any concerns, issues, accomplishments, and critical incidents as well as any unit news or individual education, or professional achievement. The last column is for unit goals established by the nurse manager and reported upon monthly and annually. These goals may include budget variance predictions, staffing issues or procedural changes.

Depicted below is a form that could be used to report monthly data:

Monthly Report

I. Financial Indicators: List any variances for line items and provide rationale for the positive or negative variance.

II. Material Issues: Describe any changes in materials or supplies, any equipment trials, or any changes in procedures requiring changes in materials.

III. Human Relations: Describe any concerns, critical incidents, issues, accomplishments, or personal and professional achievements.

IV. Unit Goals: Describe accomplishments toward your established unit goals and provide data on your progress.

Directions: Use the data in the following case study to complete the monthly report:

Susan is the nurse manager for a 46-bed general surgical unit in Palm Harbor, Florida. Susan has just received her revenue and expense report for the month. She has been speaking with the chief financial officer (CFO) about the possibility of receiving bi-weekly revenue and expense reports because she feels that problems cannot be corrected quickly with such a delay in reporting. In response, the CFO is working out the mechanics to issue reports every two weeks to help managers react more quickly to fiscal issues. (See below for revenue and expense report). Susan is also test piloting new syringes on her unit, and Kam, an RN on 7-3, has streamlined the procedure for collecting and sending specimens to the laboratory. Susan has been tracking the unit's critical incidents and discovers three medication errors for the same nurse within a two-week period. Sally, an R.N. on 3–11 has just completed an RN-BSN program, and Ron, an R.N. ,has just passed a certification exam. Susan's unit goals were to stay within 2% of budget, to assist nurses to continue their education through certification, continuing education or formal education; and to analyze the activities that could be completed by nursing assistants to decrease their down time.

Cost Center: 611 General Surgery   **Report For June 1995**

| This Month | | | Account | Year to Date | | |
Actual	Budget	Variance	Number/Description	Actual	Budget	Variance
			311.Revenue			
(371,026)	(365,800)	5,226	0110 Routine	(3,244,410)	(3,221,400)	23,010
(2,987)	(3,153)	(166)	020 Other	(27,590)	(27,768)	(178)
(374,013)	(368,953)	5,060	Total Operating Rev	(3,272,000)	(3,249,168)	22,832
			411.Salary Expense			
85,115	85,127	12	010 Salaries-Regular	730,881	749,665	18,784
2,758	0	(2,758)	020 Salaries-Per Diem	2,758	0	(2,758)
3,209	4,101	892	030 Salaries-Overtime	40,128	36,115	(4,013)
10,885	11,220	335	040 Salaries Differential	97,995	98,810	815
7,168	7,066	(102)	050 FICA	61,285	62,222	937
7,235	7,363	128	060 Health Insurance	62,125	64,846	2,721
2,212	2,358	146	070 Pension	19,855	20,766	911
1,896	1,915	19	080 Other	17,228	16,868	(360)
120,478	119,150	(1,328)	Total Salary Expense	1,032,255	1,049,292	17,037
			611.Supply Expense			
4,976	4,084	(892)	010 Patient Care Supplies	41,692	35,961	(5,731)
118	202	84	020 Office Supplies	1,097	1,780	683
371	366	(5)	030 Forms	3,111	3,224	113
0	127	127	040 Supplies Purchased	1,210	1,122	(88)

This Month			Account	Year to Date		
Actual	Budget	Variance	Number/Description	Actual	Budget	Variance
250	191	(59)	050 Equipment	1,553	1,683	130
125	149	24	060 Seminars/Meetings	1,163	1,309	146
25	17	(8)	070 Books	145	150	5
0	112	112	080 Equipment Rental	385	987	602
31	64	33	090 Miscellaneous	388	561	173
5,896	5,312	(584)	Total Supply Expense	50,744	46,777	(3,967)
			911.Interdepartmental Expense			
934	921	(13)	010 Central Supply	7,828	8,114	286
1,137	1,121	(16)	020 Pharmacy	9,527	9,868	341
1,915	1,888	(27)	030 Linen/Laundry	16,046	16,628	582
105	297	192	040 Maintenance	977	2,618	1,641
211	212	1	060 Telephone	1,962	1,870	(92)
0	21	21	070 Photocopy	124	187	63
0	13	13	090 Miscellaneous	165	112	(53)
4,302	4,473	171	Total Interdepartmental Expense	36,629	39,397	2,768
130,676	128,935	(1,741)	Total Operating Expense	1,119,628	1,135,466	15,838
(243,337)	(240,018)	3,319	Contributions from Operations	(2,152,372)	(2,113,702)	38,670
65.1%	65.1%		Contributions % of Revenue	65.8%	65.1%	

Budgeting Exercise

Introduction: It is important to have a basic understanding of budgeting and financial management as a clinical nurse. This section will provide definitions of terms, provide simple calculations, and then provide answers to the calculations.

I. A unit of service is a measurement that describes an activity in an organization. The units of service are what determine the revenue or income of the organization and describe the needed resources to offer the service.

The following definitions are basic to budgeting and financial calculations:

Beds = number of beds available for occupancy

Census = number of clients occupying beds at a specific time of day (usually midnight)

Percent occupancy = census divided by beds available x 100

Patient day = one client occupying one bed for one day

Average daily census (ADC) = patient days in a given time period divided by the number of days in the time period

Average length of stay (ALOS) = client days in a given time period divided by number of discharges in the time period.

(Definitions and budgeting calcations were taken from Finkler, S.A. (1992). *Budgeting Concepts for Nurse Managers,* Philadelphia: W.B. Saunders Co.)

II. How do client classification systems work? Classification systems are based on instruments that reflect critical indicators of care requirements. Based on the absence or presence of indicators, clients are assigned a score. Below is a printout of a classification:

Client Type	Required Care Hours in 24 Hours		Relative Value
	Range	Average	
1	0.5-2.9	2.0	0.4
2	3.0-6.9	5.0	1.0
3	7.0-15.4	10.0	2.0
4	15.5-24.0	22.0	4.4

In this example, the patient type is simply a descriptor of the classification categories. A Type 1 patient has the least workload requirements, and a Type 4 the most. The range indicates the amount of care required, and the average is the assigned value of care for all Type 1 patients. The relative value scale puts the hours of care required for each type of patient in a workload measure. Type 2 patients are arbitrarily assigned a workload value of 1.0 taking 5 hours on the average of care; and Type 3, therefore, are assigned a double workload factor because of the 10 average hours of care required.

III. How are acuity levels calculated? Listed below is a census of 18 patients with patient types identified. The calculation for acuity level is workload divided by census = acuity.
(24.0 divided by 18 = 1.33).

Client Type	Number of Clients	Relative Value	Workload
1	4	0.4	1.6
2	8	1.0	8.0
3	5	2.0	10.0
4	1	4.4	4.4
Total	18		24.0

What would the average acuity level be for this population? The calculation for average acuity is workload divided by census = acuity (120.0 divided by 18 = 6.67).

Client Type	Required Average in 24 Hours	Number of Clients	Workload
1	2.0	4	8.0
2	5.0	8	40.0
3	10.0	5	50.0
4	22.0	1	22.0
Total		18	120.0

Employers frequently discuss the terms FTEs (full-time equivalent employees) and positions or position control. These are common terms used to discuss the manpower needs of a unit or an organization. Most organizations hire at least 60–80% of their workforce with full-time equivalent employees. A full-time equivalent in hours per year = 2080. A full-time equivalent per week = 40 hours. Job positions that the unit/organization has or will hire are part-time, full-time, or per diem. Each unit is allocated a number of full-time and part-time positions which is then referred to in some institutions as a position control. The position control, or number of full-time, part-time, and per diem employees, is allocated as well as the type (registered nurse, licensed practical nurse, nurses aide) that they are permitted to hire to cover the workload of the unit.

LEARNING RESOURCES

Discussion Questions

1. Describe the three different types of budgets — zero-based, performance, and traditional.
2. Discuss how acuity levels are calculated, and workload needs are determined.
3. What is the nurse's role in providing high quality healthcare and containing costs for the organization?
4. What is the difference between a cash, a capital, and an expense budget?
5. Should nurses concern themselves with costing out nursing care? If so, why? If not, why not?

Study Questions

Matching: Write the letter of the correct response in front of each term.

____ 1. Budget	A. a form of budgeting where the whole budget is built from scratch
____ 2. Expenses	
____ 3. Strategic Planning	
____ 4. Revenues	
____ 5. Cash Budget	B. a form of budgeting where baseline data for the budget is determined from previous costs plus an inflation factor
____ 6. Capital Budget	
____ 7. Expense Budget	
____ 8. Indirect Costs	
____ 9. Traditional Budget	C. expenses related to overhead, administration, or building
____ 10. Zero-based Budget	

D. income for the provision of services

E. a financial plan that guides resource use

F. costs incurred for services provided

G. formulation of strategy for the organization

H. indicates receipts and disbursements

I. indicates major purchases of $500 or more

J. indicates payment of wages, benefits, and maintenance

SUPPLEMENTAL READINGS

Sengin, K.K. & Dreisbach, A.M. (1995). Managing with precision: A budgetary decision support model. *Journal of Nursing Administration, 25*(2), 33-44.

Shamian, J., Hagen, B., & Fogarty, T. (1994). The relationship between length of stay and required nursing care hours. *Journal of Nursing Administration, 24*(7/8).

Chapter 10

Organizational Culture and Environment

STUDY FOCUS

Assessing organizational culture is an important aspect of a nurse's role. Gaining an appreciation of cultural influences will improve a nurse's effectiveness by providing information about the interpersonal and political work environment. There are four viewpoints used when thinking about organizations — structural, human resource, political, and symbolic. A structural viewpoint focuses on the structure, roles, and relationships in organizations. The human resource perspective emphasizes the role, function, and integration of employees in the organization. A political view focuses on the allocation and distribution of constrained resources. In a symbolic view, those items that are not explained rationally are examined and meaning is attached to the situation.

Each organization has rituals, traditions, values, rules, and a structural component. Those shared beliefs, values, and practices that exist in an organization are organizational culture. Those perceptions that individuals hold about the environment are the organizational climate. Organizational culture is a more complex phenomena. It often is subtle and is not controlled by management. Management may influence culture by providing rewards and penalties, but culture is formed by a group to control its environment and to ensure safety and survival. Organizational culture serves four major functions. The first is to provide a sense of identity for group members. Secondly, it promotes a sense of commitment to the group. The third function is to enhance the stability of the group environment. Finally, it helps the group to make behavior understandable.

Several elements comprise the culture of organizations including stories, myths, rituals, and ceremonies, as well as metaphors and analogies. These elements provide concrete examples, guidance, and communication for a culture. Stories often describe heroes or conflicts. Myths are rich descriptions of events that pro-

vide inspiration and enhance belief. Rituals are embedded customs that socialize new members, provide clear messages to members, and stabilize the culture. Ceremonies entail pomp and circumstance and are functions that benefit members and the group. Metaphors and analogies are used to explain complex phenomena by simplifying the explanation using information the member knows.

The three levels of culture are the visible level, which includes physical space and social surroundings, the values of the culture, and the basic underlying assumptions that guide behavior.

Five critical elements of culture in an organization include the mission statement, formal structure, informal structure, political structure, and financial structure. Each of these five elements is critical in understanding how an organization functions.

Culture can be implicit or explicit. An explicit culture is more formal with rules, policies, and procedures clearly written and communicated. Norms and values are established. Implicit culture, on the other hand, is subtle and difficult to identify. Knowledge is not verbally shared; there are informal work rules; and people do not openly communicate their values and traditions. How then, can a nurse identify the culture on a unit? A cultural check list is a beneficial tool to analyze organizational culture. The check list should include the following: image, deportment, status symbol and reward systems, subcultures, environment and ambiance, communication, meetings, rites, rituals, and ceremonies, and sacred cows. Assessing an organizational culture is an important first step in understanding how the organization functions. Once an analysis is completed, a nurse may choose to change or build the culture to incorporate positive values and beliefs. The strategies for building culture emphasize a basic framework of support. The first step is to start building from wherever the group is currently and to work from there. Establish personal contact; use all communication channels; and facilitate open dialogue and discussion with the group. Identify shared values and goals so the focus and desired outcome are clear. Determine strategies jointly, and take action.

Positive work group cultures are important for nurse satisfaction and retention. Clinical nurses can work together to build networks and support systems for enhancing positive work environments and tackling thorny issues. Building positive cultures increases productivity and morale while improving quality client care.

LEARNING TOOLS

Group Activity: Organizational Culture Analysis

Purpose: To examine the unit where you wish to practice when you complete your educational requirements. Use the following Organizational Culture Check List to analyze the organization (the check list has been adapted from the Huber text).

ORGANIZATIONAL CULTURE CHECK LIST

Aspects of Culture	Questions for Assessment
1. Image	How do the nurses dress? Casually or Formally? What symbols or slogans are used? Is the unit aesthetically pleasing?
2. Deportment	What is the level of courtesy shown to clients' families? Are males and females treated equally? Are all healthcare workers treated with respect?
3. Status Symbols	Are the nurses' parking and lounges comparable to physicians' and administrators'? Is there an elitist attitude? If so by whom? Are offices and equipment comparable?
4. Subcultures	Do nurses from the same cultural background tend to form friendships with each other more easily? Are there cliques on the unit? Are new employees welcomed by the group?
5. Environment and Ambiance	How well is the physical structure maintained? Is the decor attractive and well kept? Is there space for classrooms and lounges? Are rooms reserved for special groups?
6. Communication	How does the CEO communicate with nurses? Does the Vice President of Nursing make rounds on all units? How does the nurse manager share information with employees? Does the important communication take place in formal meetings or informally in groups?
7. Meetings	Who participates in what meetings? How are participants for meetings selected? How are decisions made in committee? Where are meetings held? Are refreshments provided?
8. Rites, Rituals, and Ceremonies	How are holidays celebrated? Is longevity recognized? What events are celebrated and recognized? What are the policies for orientation and termination?
9. Sacred Cows	Who are the heroes/heroines? What subjects are taboo? Are there policies that are untouchable?

The information you gather from your cultural assessment will provide you with a basic understanding of the organization's culture. You will be able to tell is the culture is explicit or implicit. You will be able to tell whether the organization is formal or informal, how policies and procedures are made, and the nature of interpersonal interactions among staff. This data will provide you with information that will be useful in determining the type of unit where you wish to work.

CASE STUDY

Susan is a registered nurse on a 58-bed neurosurgical unit for a large community hospital in Portland, Oregon. She is working on a project concerning organizational cultural assessments as part of the requirements for her Master's Degree in Nursing. Susan has discovered tension among the staff about their new roles after an organizational redesign. There is much resistance on the part of the staff members about "letting go" of their old responsibilities and taking new ones. Susan carefully examines the written communications including memos, policies, procedures, and job descriptions. She notices that many of the documents have not changed since the organizational redesign. Traditionally, the hospital has relied heavily on written documents to provide stability and guidance for the staff. Now, staff are feeling insecure and reluctant to change. What should Susan do? *Assess* *Open discussion* *Communicate* *Determine some strategies* *Implement plans*

Case Study Questions

1. Has the organizational culture where Susan works been <u>explicit</u> or implicit? *They go things in writing (Policies and Procedures)*
2. What organizational viewpoint is most evident in this culture? *Structure*
3. What strategies should Susan take to realign the organizational culture? *Start where group is*
4. What critical cultural elements must Susan examine?

LEARNING RESOURCES

Discussion Questions

1. To do an in-depth cultural assessment of an organization, how long would it take, and what criteria would you use to evaluate the organization?
2. What strategies could a nurse employ to change or build organizational culture?
3. What is the nurse's role in building organizational culture?

4. What is the difference between implicit and explicit culture? Which type of culture is easier to analyze?
5. What are the critical cultural elements in an organization, and how do they strengthen the existing organizational culture?

Study Questions

Multiple Choice: Circle the correct response.

1. Susan, an R.N. on the neurosurgical unit, is assessing organizational manifestations by cultural level. When she assesses the visible level, what is Susan examining?
   A. the balance of cost, quality, and access to care
   B. the physical space and social environment
   C. the guidelines of the organization
   D. the values of what ought to be in the organization

2. After Susan examines the cultural levels, she begins examining the five critical cultural elements in the organization. What five elements does she examine?
   A. values, mission statement, basic assumptions, and formal and informal structure
   B. mission statement, basic assumptions, and formal, informal, and political structures
   C. values, basic assumption, and formal, informal, and political structures
   D. mission statement, and formal, informal, political, and financial structures

3. Susan knows that an organization needs a framework of support for building a culture. Which of the following are necessary components for supporting a culture?
   A. values, communication, actions, and strategies
   B. communication, values, strategies, and mission statement
   C. actions, strategies, mission statement, and shared values
   D. mission statement, strategies, actions, and communication

4. Susan decides to take a structural view of the organization in her cultural analysis. What data should she collect?
   A. data on the allocation and distribution of scarce resources
   B. existing symbols and signs in the organization
   C. the communication and interpersonal network in the organization
   D. the formal roles, relationships, and organizational structures

5. Susan is teaching a continuing education class on organizational culture. Which of the following definitions should she use to define organizational culture?
   - A. shared beliefs, values, and assumptions that exist in an organization
   - B. perceptions that individuals have about the environment in the organization
   - C. Culture gives meaning and significance to activities in organizations.
   - D. Every organization has values, rituals, and rules.

SUPPLEMENTAL READINGS

Coeling, H.V. & Simms, L.M. (1993). Facilitating innovation at the nursing unit level through cultural assessment, Part 1: How to keep management ideas from falling on deaf ears. *Journal of Nursing Administration, 23*(4), 46-53.

Coeling, H.V. & Simms, L.M. (1993). Facilitating innovation at the unit level through cultural assessment, Part 2: Adapting managerial ideas to the unit work group. *Journal of Nursing Administration, 23*(5), 13-20.

McDaniel, C. & Stumpf, L. (1993). The organizational culture: Implications for nursing service. *Journal of Nursing Administration, 23*(4), 54-60.

Sovie, M.D. (1993). Hospital culture — Why create one? *Nursing Economics, 11*(2), 69-90.

Chapter 11

Organizations, Mission Statements, Policies, and Procedures

STUDY FOCUS

Organizations are composed of a group of individuals who each have specific responsibilities to act together toward the goals of the organization. Organizational structure is provided by management to efficiently and effectively meet organizational goals and to provide direction to employees, vendors, and consumers. Healthcare organizations are complex and require professional staff to accomplish their mission. The mission statement of the organization describes the product; for healthcare organizations the product is client care.

Organizations are social systems comprised of the environment and individuals. The environment is composed of the internal and external environments, roles, and goals or expectations. Individuals have their own needs, personalities, and personal agendas. At times individuals' needs or desires may be in conflict with organizational goals. By accepting employment within an organization, employees infer that they will abide by the organizational philosophy.

Organizations have mission statements to guide the institution and provide direction to employees. Mission statements are composed of a philosophy, a purpose, and objectives. A philosophy is a statement of values and beliefs. It is abstract, describing a vision and providing guidance. The nursing department's philosophy should be congruent with the organizational philosophy and include the three vital components of client, nurse, and nursing practice. The purpose of the organization is its reason for existence. It spells out the service(s) to be provided. The nursing purpose must take into consideration the organization's purpose, the state Nurse Practice Act, and legal concerns. The objectives are hoped for outcomes directing activities toward organizational goal accomplishment. Objectives must be behaviorally specific statements in written format. They must be realistic, attainable, and priority-focused.

Policies and procedures are written to clearly articulate the rules of the organization that are derived from the mission statement. Policies and procedures are developed to coordinate the work of the organization. Policies are general guidelines that speak to repetitive problems or tasks in the organization. The policies help coordinate plans, control performance, and increase the consistency of activities. Policies are usually written, although informal policies may exist. Policies speak to all employees and not just one job category. Procedures provide a step-by-step plan to complete a task. They are developed for those activities that recur on a regular basis, and they provide a performance guideline for them. Procedures are written, provide a reference, and are typically in a consistent format. The procedure format includes the purpose of the activity, the individual who is responsible for performing the activity, steps in the procedure, and supplies or equipment necessary to accomplish the task.

A positive work environment fostered by a philosophy that espouses group participation and commitment is paramount to a successful, effective team. A caring approach that focuses on common elements of successful organizations, that retains employees, and that includes a managerial commitment to employees, strong leadership, and competitive salaries and benefits fosters employee commitment. A value of caring and excellence for all constituents, clients, staff, and other healthcare workers enhances work commitment and quality outcomes. Support for autonomy, innovation, and risk taking is embedded in a team-building philosophy. In contrast, behaviors that create barriers to organizational excellence include telling versus asking people about their needs, depersonalizing members of the organization, acting without habitual courtesy, and showing contempt for individuals. These behaviors are exhibited by preferential treatment, insensitivity, a lack of communication, ambiguity in job requirements, and a user attitude toward employees.

LEARNING TOOLS

Role Play #1

Caring Behaviors That Build Teams and Promote Commitment

Character One = Jill is the Vice President of Nursing and frequently makes rounds on all 15 client care units in the hospital. Jill is supportive of all her staff and empowers them to make autonomous decisions. Frequently clinical and administrative staff consult with her on their projects.

Character Two = Jack is a clinical nurse who was hired three months previously and has been doing an outstanding job with clients, but he is having some problems interacting with residents.

Character Three = Joe is a resident and has just started working with one of Jack's clients. Joe has been at the hospital for one year and has been short with staff on occasions.

Character Four = Sally is a nurse's aide who is working with Jack to provide supportive care to the clients.

✦   ✦   ✦   ✦

Jill is rounding on all the units when she hears voices beginning to rise. She turns the corner to see Joe, Sally, and Jack discussing a problem in loud voices.

Role-play Questions:

1. What should Jill do? Should she intervene? If so, what should she say?
2. What strategies could she employ using a caring approach to intervene?
3. How can she manage the situation to empower all of the individuals involved?

Role-play Worksheet

CHARACTERS	STUDENT ASSIGNED
Jill, The Vice President of Nursing	_____
Joe, the Resident	_____
Sally, the Nurse's Aide	_____
Jack, the Clinical Nurse	_____

Which character have you been assigned?

What are your character's goals in this situation?

How can the other characters assist you in achieving your goals?

What might the other characters do to hinder you in achieving your goals?

What strategies and probes do you plan to use in this situation?

Role Play #2

Behaviors that Create Barriers to Organizational Excellence

Using the same characters (Jill, Joe, Jack, and Sally) and the same scenario (Jill rounds the corner to discover a problem), role-play a situation using contempt behaviors which block effectiveness and increase turnover.

Role-play Questions:

1. What should Jill do? Should she intervene? If so, what should she say?
2. What strategies could she employ to create a barrier and disempower employees?
3. Discuss why individuals choose to use contempt behaviors to resolve problems.

Role-play Worksheet

CHARACTERS	STUDENT ASSIGNED
Jill, The Vice President of Nursing	_____
Joe, the Resident	_____
Sally, the Nurses Aide	_____
Jack, the Clinical Nurse	_____

Which character have you been assigned?

What are your character's goals in this situation?

How can the other characters assist you in achieving your goals?

What might the other characters do to hinder you in achieving your goals?

What strategies and probes do you plan to use in this situation?

CASE STUDY

Jacqueline is a newly hired Vice President of Nursing for a 250-bed hospital in Maine. She has carefully read the mission statement of the organization and decides to make rounds on the units to see how integrated it is on the units. The mission statement describes the hospital as a community-based center of excellence that provides care to all clients in a cost-effective manner. On her rounds, she stops to talk with Debbie and Karen, both of whom are nurse managers. She asks them what the mission of the organization is, and Debbie replies that it is to provide high-quality healthcare, and Karen says that it is to increase the market share for obstetrics patients. Jacqueline also asks several staff nurses about the mission statement and gets a variety of responses.

Case Study Questions

1. What purpose does a mission statement serve?
2. Is it a problem that nurse managers and clinical nurses are unable to recite or explain the mission statement?
3. What can Jacqueline do to increase employee awareness of the mission statement?

LEARNING RESOURCES

Discussion Questions

1. What are the differences between a philosophy, a purpose, and an objective?
2. How does the organizational philosophy relate to the nursing philosophy?
3. Are employees obliged to agree with or carry out the mission statement? If so, why?
4. How can nurse leaders promote positive work cultures?
5. What is the clinical nurse's role in developing philosophy, purpose, and objectives?

Study Questions

True and False: Circle the correct answer.

T F 1. An organization has a purpose, structure, and individuals.

T F 2. A philosophy describes the reason the organization exists.

T F 3. The purpose relates the values and beliefs of the organization.

T F 4. Objectives are outcomes that direct an activity toward goal accomplishment.

T F 5. The three core components of a nursing philosophy are the client, the nurse, and the physician. *← procedure*

T F 6. A policy is a step-by-step guide to solve common problems.

T F 7. A procedure is a general guideline that guides goal accomplishment.

T F 8. Caring philosophies empower individuals and assist in organizational goal attainment.

T F 9. Contempt behaviors create barriers to excellence in organizations.

T F 10. Nurses desire improvements in image, autonomy, and collaboration.

SUPPLEMENTAL READINGS

Graham, P., Constantini, S., Balik, B., Bedfore, B., Hooke, M., Papin, D., Quamme, M; & Rivard, R. (1987). Operationalizing a nursing philosophy. *Journal of Nursing Administration, 17*(3), 14-18.

Nyberg, J. (1993). Teaching caring to the nurse administrator. *Journal of Nursing Administration, 23*(1), 11-17.

Chapter 12

Organizational Structure: Concepts

STUDY FOCUS

Organizational structure is essential for the efficient and effective management of work, power, and control in organizations. The structure of an organization is the way in which personnel are divided by their tasks and coordinated to accomplish organizational goals. Many factors are examined before organizational structures are designed. These factors include the age of an organization, its size, technology, internal and external environment, and its resources. There is both formal and informal organizational structure. Formal structure refers to what is clearly written into an organizational chart. Informal structure is the internal and external network of relationships and interdependencies around the organization. One aspect of the informal structure is the "grapevine."

Important concepts of management are associated with structure such as division of labor, span of control, scalar process, and line and staff positions. The division of labor refers to the assignment and distribution of the organization's work to individuals who have the authority and responsibility to complete the job. The span of control refers to the number of subordinates one manager oversees. The scalar process is the levels within the organization. Line positions are those that are in direct line of hierarchical authority and central to producing a product of the organization. On the other hand, staff positions provide the expertise and knowledge to meet organizational goals.

Mintzberg (1983) has identified technology, social environment, size, and task repetitiveness as major influences on structure. In healthcare, sophisticated technologies; rapid, complex decisions; and the changing professional workforce present a formidable challenge for administrators and require decentralized, autonomous teams working to promote quality client care. Organizational size changes as it ages. An organization begins with a small, organic, and unelaborate structure. The second stage is entrepreneurially directed by a dynamic, powerful executive. A formalized structure emerges, and a bureaucracy begins to form. As the organization ages and grows, divisional structures develop, and finally, it may shift to a matrix structure.

Mintzberg (1983) identifies five basic structural designs: the simple structure, machine bureaucracy, professional bureaucracy, divisionalized form, and adhocracy. Mintzberg also addresses the basic coordinating mechanisms to accomplish work. They are mutual adjustment, direct supervision, standardization of work processes, standardization of work outputs, and standardization of worker skills. The more complex the environment, the more fluid and autonomous it is, needing little supervision.

Structures can be flat or tall. Tall structures are typically in a pyramid shape with the Board of Control at the top and the staff at the bottom. Board members typically control fiscal resources and make policy. Within each level of the pyramid, there are job positions. Each job is a group of tasks that is performed by an individual. Each position carries with it a degree of authority, accountability, and responsibility. Authority is the right to act or direct others. Accountability is the liability of task performance, and responsibility is the assignment and acceptance of a task. Organizations may be centralized or decentralized. Centralized organizations have board members and administrators with power and authority at the top of the organization. Decentralized organizations are just the opposite. They empower staff at all levels to make decisions and solve pressing problems. Decentralized organizations usually have flat structures with few hierarchical levels.

In turbulent environments, such as healthcare, decentralized structures are efficient and effective because they respond rapidly to environmental change. Nurse administrators must continually examine the structure and process in order to manage resources effectively and expedite the work of the organization. One method of modifying the structure is called restructuring. Restructuring is modifying the existing structural components of an organization; whereas, reengineering, another method, is a renovation of the processes used to accomplish goals. Changing the structure of nursing organizations is essential to stay competitive and provide community-based care to clients through integrated healthcare systems.

LEARNING TOOLS

Group Activity: Understanding Organizational Structure

Purpose: To gain a clear understanding of the purpose and function of organizational structures.

Directions: Discuss the importance of organizational structure for work, power, and control elements. Structure creates an environment in which practice takes place. Describe nursing administrators', nurse managers', and clinical nurses' roles in changing the organizational structure to improve client outcomes. What type of an organizational structure works best in a turbulent, changing healthcare environment? Describe activities nurses can use to create a positive work environment.

CASE STUDY

Jo is a nurse manager of a 45-bed surgical unit with a position control of 58 FTEs, and which currently employs 65 individuals. Christa is the nurse educator assigned to the surgical unit. Christa works with all of the surgical units since she is a clinical nurse specialist whose focus is surgical care. Jo and Christa work well as a team, and they establish annual goals together and meet monthly to review progress. Jo's task is to be responsible for the fiscal and human resource management, and Christa's responsibilities include the education of new and existing employees.

Case Study Questions

1. Is Jo in a line or staff position? Is Christa in a line or staff position? What is the difference between line and staff positions?
2. For what tasks is Jo held accountable? For what tasks is Christa held accountable?
3. Who has the authority to make decisions for the surgical unit?
4. Which resources can Jo and Christa consult to determine their level of accountability?

LEARNING RESOURCES

Discussion Questions

1. In turbulent environments, is a centralized or decentralized structure best for accomplishing the work of the organization? Provide a rationale for your answer.
2. What are some methods nurse administrators can use to change the structure in order to deliver high quality care to clients?

3. Describe the five basic coordinating mechanisms that organizations use to coordinate their work.
4. What is the role of the board in an organization? How can clinical nurses impact board level decisions?
5. What is the difference between restructuring and reengineering? Give an example of each.

Study Questions

Matching: Write the letter of the correct response in front of each term.

I	1.	Line position
C	2.	Staff position
D	3.	Authority
E	4.	Accountability
F	5.	Responsibility
A	6.	Scalar process
B	7.	Span of control
J	8.	Reengineering
G	9.	Centralized
H	10.	Decentralized

A. the creation of levels of authority in a hierarchy

B. the number of workers supervised by a manager

C. a position that provides expertise and knowledge for accomplishing organizational goals

D. the right to act or direct others

E. the liability associated with task performance

F. the allocation or acceptance of tasks

G. when the power to make decisions is concentrated at the top of an organization

H. when the power to make decisions is filtered down toward the individual worker

I. direct line of hierarchical authority

J. changing the operational process of an organization

SUPPLEMENTAL READINGS

Hall, G., Rosenthal, J., & Wade, J. (l993). How to make reengineering really work. *Harvard Business Review, 71*(6), 119-131.

Manthey, M. & Miller, D. (1994). Empowerment through levels of authority. *Journal of Nursing Administration, 24*(7/8), 23.

Mintzberg, H. (1983). *Structure in fives: Designing effective organizations.* Englewood Cliffs, NJ: Prentice-Hall.

Chapter 13

Organizational Structure: Types

STUDY FOCUS

In the past, the healthcare service industry has not operated as a business. Today, healthcare is big business and must be responsive to cost and quality issues and changing reimbursement patterns. Organizational structures are one mechanism that provides a framework for the division of labor and the accomplishment of work. The three types of organizations are bureaucracy, matrix, and adhocracy. These organizational types can be viewed on a continuum with the classic bureaucracy on one end and the delegated organizational type adhocracy on the opposite end.

A bureaucracy is a tall, pyramidal, hierarchical structure where the power is centralized at the top. In a pyramidal structure, the decision makers are at the top, and the workers are at the bottom. Line positions are those that are in the chain of command and who directly contribute to the product or service of the organization. The strategic apex is another term used to denote the top decision maker positions. The operating core are the workers and the middle line managers coordinating the work. Technocrats are individuals who design, plan, change, or train people to do the work. Support staff provide services to enhance the technocrats productivity.

A matrix structure is used for complex work environments. It is a combination of bureaucracy and project teams. In a matrix structure, single individuals may report to two or more individuals and be evaluated by them on specific components of their work. This structure is a complicated one which requires coordination and careful evaluation. The advantages include maximizing the use of specialists and interdisciplinary team work. Its disadvantages include the need for time consuming activities such as monitoring and evaluating multiple project teams and individuals and for ensuring optimal productivity from groups.

Adhocracies are used when highly specialized professional groups practice together. Little supervision is needed, and individual workers are assigned to project teams to complete work.

There are five basic organizational types ranging from the most simple to the more complex type. The simple structure has a wide span of control, minimal or no middle line, and no staff. The organization is typically small and new with few guidelines. A machine bureaucracy is an elaborate structure of administrative and support personnel, large units, and a pyramidal hierarchy. A professional bureaucracy has a flat structure, with few midlevel managers, but a large support staff to assist professional workers. A divisionalized form is a collection of quasi-autonomous units with a central administration. An adhocracy is a highly organic form composed of professional workers who elect to manage themselves and a flat administrative structure.

An organizational chart is used to graphically display the formal structure for an organization. The formal structure depicts the formal communication channels — who reports to whom and the levels of authority. The informal structure is a network within an organization that is typically oral in nature, and composed of friends and co-workers who share information. The organizational chart depicts vertical or horizontal structures. Vertical structures show how tall or centralized an organization is, and horizontal structures refer to flat or decentralized organizations.

Nursing leaders are faced with a complex, turbulent, and constantly changing healthcare environment to manage. They are challenged to respond to client needs and healthcare issues. Four major leadership initiatives to cope with healthcare changes are downsizing management, decentralizing support services, centralizing supply distribution, and organizing labor around technology.

Nurses who lead their organizations to success will also use new or reconfigured hospital structures. The trends noted by responsive leadership teams are flattened organizations, fluid structures, outcomes orientation, redefined staff functions with managerial accountability, reduced staff costs, subcontracting services, and refocusing on the core business. Work design, restructuring, and reengineering are all strategies to reposition a healthcare agency in a competitive manner. Layoffs, downsizing, and substitution of assistants for RNs are only short-term solutions for the cost concerns of managers. Nursing leaders must take a proactive stance and provide a vision for the organization, one that combines cost and quality into an efficient, effective healthcare system that is grounded in positive client outcomes.

LEARNING TOOLS

Group Activity: Organizational Chart Analysis

Purpose: To analyze an organizational chart in order to determine the channels of communication, staff and line positions, centralized versus decentralized structure, and a pyramidal or flat structure.

Directions:

Questions

1. Is this a pyramidal or flat organizational structure?
2. Are communication channels simple or complex?
3. Are there any staff positions? If so, what are they?
4. How many levels are in the hierarchy?
5. Is this a centralized or a decentralized chart?

(See page 46 for answers to the above questions.)

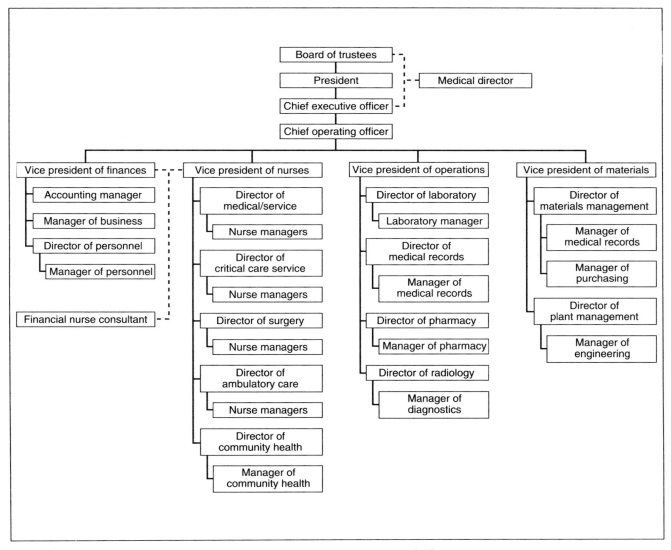

Figure 1. Hospital Organizational Chart

Hospital Organizational Chart Answers:
   This is a pyramidal organizational structure with seven levels in the hierarchy. The communication channels are complex with a detailed reporting structure. It appears to be a very centralized organizational structure because of the multiple levels. There are two identified staff positions, the medical director and the financial nurse consultant.)

CASE STUDY

Sylvia is a vice president of a 720-bed acute care facility in New York. The hospital has been having severe financial problems because of the changes in reimbursement. Sylvia has met with the Chief Executive Officer (CEO) and the Chief Financial Officer (CFO) who both want immediate action to get the bottom line in the black. Since Sylvia has the largest budget with the largest number of FTEs she is asked to make all the cuts in her department. The CEO and CFO suggested layoffs, hiring assistive unlicensed personnel (UAP), and merging units to decrease the number of nurse managers in the hospital. They are not telling Sylvia what to do, however. If she can think of other cost cutting strategies, she is free to use them. (Sylvia leaves the meeting rather somber.)

Case Study Questions

1. What should Sylvia do?
2. Will the suggestions that the CEO and CFO made solve all Sylvia's problems and save money for the hospital?
3. Are the suggestions that the CEO and CFO made long-term or short-term strategies?
4. What other strategies could be employed to cut costs?

LEARNING RESOURCES

Discussion Questions

1. Are there differences between the healthcare service industry and the private business sector?
2. What type of organizational structure would be best for a highly complex, turbulent, healthcare environment that employes specialists?
3. What is the difference between centralized and decentralized organizations?
4. Describe the difference between a line and a staff position. Provide an example of each.
5. When would a matrix structure for an organization be useful? What are the advantages and disadvantages of a matrix structure?

Study Questions

Matching: Write the letter of the correct response in front of each term.

I	1.	Bureaucracy
H	2.	Matrix
J	3.	Adhocracy
G	4.	Pyramidal
F	5.	Technostructure
E	6.	Support staff
D	7.	Operating core
C	8.	Horizontal structure
B	9.	Machine bureaucracy
A	10.	Divisionalized form

A. a collection of semiautonomous units linked by a central administrative structure

B. a large administrative and support staff and a tall hierarchy

C. few administrative layers between top administrators and workers

D. those who perform the work of the organization by providing the service

E. individuals who perform activities that enable individuals to do the direct work of the organization

F. analysts who design, plan, change, or train people to do the work of the organization

G. tall, shaped with a wide base and narrow apex

H. a complex combination of a hierarchical structure with project teams

I. tall, hierarchical, centralized structure

J. flat, decentralized structure with project teams

SUPPLEMENTAL READINGS

Burns, L. & Thorpe, D. (1993). Trends and models in physician hospital organization. *Health Care Management Review, 18*(4), 7-20.

Dumaine, B. (1993). Payoff from the new management. *Fortune, 128*(15), 103-110.

Nagelkerk, J. & Henry, B. (1993). Chain reaction. *Graduating Nurse,* 19-23.

Chapter 14

Decentralization and Shared Governance

STUDY FOCUS

Decision-making authority in an organization is an essential component of job and professional autonomy. Decision-making power can be centralized with a few administrators at the top or decentralized, passing the power on to the individuals that the decision affects directly. Centralization and decentralization can be ranges on a continuum with centralization at one end and decentralization at the opposite extreme. Decisions can be viewed as either more or less centralized or decentralized. There is rarely a situation in which all decisions are exclusively centralized or exclusively decentralized. Vertical decentralization is the distribution of formal power down the chain of command, and horizontal decentralization is the distribution of formal power outside the chain of command where support staff participate in the decision-making process. (When an administration centralizes the structure, they are controlling decision making and holding power at the top of the organization. In contrast, an administration that decentralizes decision making empowers employees at all levels of the organization to participate.)

During turbulent times, in complex environments, and with professional staff, decentralization is a useful tool to ensure that the organization stays flexible, innovative, and committed to solving complex, multidisciplinary problems. Participation in decision making at all levels fosters autonomy, accountability, and worker responsibility.

Communication to and from individuals is extremely important in decentralized organizations. Nurse administrators are experimenting with many different models of participatory decision making to empower nurses to provide quality care to clients. Shared governance is one professional practice framework that espouses an accountability-based governance structure. Shared governance is a system that fosters creativity and flexibility by empowering nurses to make autonomous clinical decisions through for-

mal processes. The major nursing service components of shared governance include practice, quality education, and peer governance.

Shared governance was first implemented in the late 1970s as a method to improve nurse satisfaction, improve retention, and enhance the recruitment of clinical nurses. Difficulties in establishing a shared governance environment commonly occur in a bureaucratic organization because of the complicated communication networks, rigid reporting structures, and elaborate policies and procedures that govern employee behavior. Another common problem in implementing shared governance is the difficulty of making a true change instead of a cosmetic or name change. It is much easier for an administration to use the terminology, but retain all authority and decision-making power.

The implementation of shared governance in an organization creates a constant tension between organizational and professional goals. Nurses exert their influence or control by clearly defining and articulating their scope and standards of practice, their nursing care delivery system, their knowledge specialization, their knowledge and resource development priorities, and their self- or peer evaluation.

Three major models of professional governance are the councilar model, the congressional model, and the administrative shared governance model. The councilar model has committees which are elected and which have clearly defined authority and function. The councilar model typically has at least one committee on each of the following: practice, education, management, and quality improvement. The congressional model includes officers and an elected cabinet. It is modeled after the national government's structure. The administrative shared governance model divides administration and clinical into two separate components and identifies the authority for each. Committees and forums are held together, and decisions are made at the level where the actual work takes place. Both the administrative and council structure have decision-making power.

Changes in healthcare delivery require responsiveness to new client care demands on an on-going basis. Clinical nurses are being held accountable for their actions and must take responsibility in designing and delivering care. Healthcare organizations will continue to change to maintain their viability and increase their marketshare, causing mergers, consolidations, multisite systems, and integrated healthcare networks. Nursing leaders are challenged to restructure roles in order to decentralize authority to the point of service, empower clinical nurses, increase multitasking, develop work processes that support client-care delivery, and design new skill mixes.

LEARNING TOOLS

Group Activity: Analysis of Organizational Structure

Purpose: To analyze an organization in order to determine if it is a centralized or decentralized organization, and to determine if a shared governance framework is established.

Directions: Select a healthcare organization that you are familiar with and answer the following questions:

a. Where is the power in the organization?

b. How much authority does each manager have?

c. Who has what decision-making responsibility?

d. How many levels of hierarchy are there in the organization?

e. Do clinical nurses make autonomous clinical decisions?

f. Are clinical nurses elected or appointed to organizational committees?

g. Do clinical nurses participate in hiring, evaluating, and scheduling decisions?

h. How are clinical nurses innovative ideas encouraged and received by administration?

i. How are assignments made on the nursing units?

After you have thought about these questions, design an organizational structure that facilitates participation. This exercise will help you determine the type of organizational structure that you are comfortable with and give you ideas about the type of work environment you will look for when seeking employment.

Remember, a more decentralized structure enables clinical nurses to participate at all levels of decision making. Communication is horizontal and vertical and innovations are encouraged.

CASE STUDY

Joyce has been a vice president of nursing at a 600-bed community hospital for fifteen years. She has established a hierarchical nursing service and decides it is time to cut out some of the unnecessary organizational layers to contain costs. Joyce announces at the monthly management meeting in May that it is imperative that nursing management downsize. She says she will be consulting with several individuals to make the best possible and least painful choices. Joyce also announces that she has developed a shared governance model and provides a handout of the committee structure for the nursing service department. Joyce directs the managers to tell the employees that they are now working in a shared government environment and to solicit volunteers for the committees. Managers should submit volunteer names to the executive secretary. The secretary will notify the appropriate committee members when problems arise and arrange for them to meet.

Case Study Questions

1. Did Joyce implement a shared governance framework?

2. How is participation in decision making encouraged at all levels in the nursing department?

3. What benefits are there to espousing a shared governance framework?

LEARNING RESOURCES

Discussion Questions

1. Discuss the disadvantages and advantages of centralized and decentralized organizational structures.

2. How do changes in healthcare influence the type of governance model a hospital will choose to implement?

3. Compare and contrast the three major types of governance models.

4. What is meant by "only a cosmetic change occurred when shared governance was implemented"?

5. What is the clinical nurse's role in a shared governance model?

Study Questions

True and False: Circle the correct answer.

T ~~F~~ 1. The congressional model uses a council format and separates the clinical and administrative tract.

T ~~F~~ 2. The administrative model elects a president and cabinet of officers who represent each nursing unit.

~~T~~ F 3. The councilar model is composed of councils with elected positions.

T ~~F~~ 4. All clinical nurses are in favor of a shared governance system where accountability and decision making are encouraged.

T ~~F~~ 5. Implementation of shared governance systems is costly and requires considerable time and effort.

~~T~~ F 6. Nurse leaders are challenged to design effective delivery systems in multihospital systems and integrated networks.

~~T~~ F 7. Centralization is the concentration of decision-making authority at the top of the organization.

~~T~~ F 8. Decentralization is the dispersment of decision-making authority throughout the organization.

T ~~F~~ 9. An organization is either centralized or decentralized.

T ~~F~~ 10. Savvy administrators will decentralize during crisis and centralize during stable times.

SUPPLEMENTAL READINGS

Evan, K., Aubry, K., Hawkins, M., Curley, T., & Porter-O'Grady, T. (1995). Whole systems shared governance: A model for the integrated health system. *Journal of Nursing Administration*, 25(5), 18-27.

Minnen, T.G., Berger, E., Ames, A., Dubree, M., Baker, W., & Spinella, J. (1993). Sustaining work redesign innovations through shared governance. *Journal of Nursing Administration*, 23(7/8), 35-40.

Moss, M. & Bailes, B. (1993). Shared governance: super units in the surgical suite. *Journal of Nursing Administration*, 58(5), 1003-1014.

Chapter 15

Delegation

STUDY FOCUS

The complexity and cost-constrained nature of the healthcare delivery system necessitates a multi-disciplinary, multilevel approach to the provision of client care. Nurses must learn to delegate effectively to coordinate multidisciplinary teams and to manage especially complex client cases. Delegation is the ability to accomplish tasks through other people while maintaining accountability. A delegator is an individual who assigns or delegates the task to another. A delegate is an individual who accepts the delegated task. To effectively delegate, the delegator must supervise the work by providing direction for task accomplishment, periodically checking on the progress, and then evaluating the outcome.

Delegation is not dumping unpleasant work on others, being bossy, or abdicating responsibility and accountability. Managers should not delegate personal accountability, the disciplining of employees, or the recognition and praise of good work to others. Delegation is used to improve others' skills, assign new tasks, build teams, and complete tasks that you do not have time to do. As a nurse, you will delegate both nursing activities, the tasks essential to provide client care, and nonnursing activities, the tasks necessary to support client care. The six basic principles of delegation are to know yourself and team members; assess the strengths, weaknesses, job description, and situation of yourself and your team members; know your state practice act; assess your job requirements; communicate clearly; and evaluate the outcome.

The four basic steps in delegating effectively include selecting a competent individual, explaining both the task and outcome anticipated, giving the authority and resources necessary to complete the task, and providing opportunity for input and evaluation. When trying to decide which tasks are appropriate to delegate, the following should be considered: the potential for harm, the complexity of the activity, the degree of problem solving and innovation required, the predictability of the outcome, and the extent of interaction necessary with clients. Carefully analyzing each task and matching it to an appropriate individual will assist in positive task accomplishment.

Many managers choose not to delegate because they need to control situations, fear the incompetence of their subordinates, have an attitude of superiority, or are concerned about poor outcomes. Subordinates may also be fearful of delegation because they lack self-confidence, fear criticism and overwork, have no incentives to complete new tasks, and like the convenience of having the boss solve the problems. Once a task is delegated, the delegator is still accountable for the outcome. Nurses must become familiar with the Nurse Practice Act for their state in order to understand the rules that govern nursing practice and provide direction on delegation. The American Nurses' Association's Code for Nurses is a handy guide for ethical problems. Nurses *must* understand the liability that is inherent in delegating activities so that they can avoid any negligence through a failure to act in accordance with established standards.

Registered nurses are challenged with the delegation of tasks to unlicensed assistive personnel (UAP). Evaluating individuals, their job description, skill level, task, and the required level of supervision they need is essential for effective delegation. Guidelines for delegating to UAP include assigning tasks that are routine and standard with outcomes that are relatively predictable and where the illness and hospitalization is not life threatening. Careful evaluation of the delegate, task, and outcome is essential for safe nursing practice. Effective use of delegation builds teams, improves an individual's skills, and enhances quality care.

LEARNING TOOLS

Role Play #1

Delegating Tasks: Exploring Roles

Character One = Jessica is a nurse manager of a 45-bed surgical unit. Jessica is supportive of her staff and facilitates their growth and development.

Character Two = Barb is a RN on the surgical unit. She has worked for three years as a RN and is well respected by the staff. She leads a team including Julie and Anna who are both nurse's aides.

Character Three = Julie, an experienced nurse's aide on the surgical unit. She enjoys client care and works well with Barb. Julie is hesitant to offer any additional assistance to Barb even though Julie knows Barb is busy, because Julie is afraid additional assistance will become expected of her, and she wants to leave the hospital exactly at 3:30 P.M., so she can pick her son up from school to prevent the additional expense of day care.

Character Four = Anna is a nurse's aide who was hired three months ago and has no previous experience beyond the training she has received at the hospital. Anna also feels that RNs should do more work than she does because they get paid more.

✦   ✦   ✦   ✦

Barb is having trouble completing her work before the 7–3 shift ends. She feels that there is not enough time in a shift to complete the required activities for safe client care. Barb becomes frustrated when she notices the nurse's aides sitting down and chatting at the desk while she provides care at an unrelenting pace. Barb approaches Jessica explaining that she is overworked, and the nurse's aides are unproductive. She requests to have another RN put on her team. Barb tells Jessica that she would be willing to give up both nurse's aides for one experienced RN. Jessica explains to Barb that there is not enough money in the budget for any more RNs and that she will have to learn to delegate her work to the nurse's aides.

Role-play Questions:

1. What process should Barb use to determine what tasks she could delegate to Anna and Julie?
2. What should she say to Anna and Julie when she delegates tasks to them? How do you think Anna and Julie will respond?
3. Can the nurse's aides refuse to take on additional work?
4. Would both nurse's aides be able to take on the same tasks?
5. How can Barb manage the situation without becoming frustrated and burned out?

Directions: Role play this scenario showing how Julie can help Barb become comfortable with delegating. Practice delegating tasks to the nurse's aides.

Role-play Worksheet

CHARACTERS	STUDENT ASSIGNED
Jessica, the nurse manager	_____
Barb, the RN	_____
Julie, the experienced nurse's aide	_____
Anna, the new nurse's aide	_____

Which character have you been assigned?

What are your character's goals in this situation?

How can the other characters assist you in achieving your goals?

What might the other characters do to hinder you in achieving your goals?

What strategies and probes do you plan to use in this situation?

CASE STUDY

Jon is a RN on the 3–11 shift for a medical unit. The nurse manager just announced that due to budget cuts, unlicensed assistive personnel (UAP) were going to be hired to assist RNs. Jon is assigned to a pod which consists of himself and two UAPs to care for 18 clients. Jon realizes he cannot complete the work himself, so he requests a description of the experience, skill level, and familiarity with the hospital that the two UAPs have. After the nurse manager provides Jon with this information, Jon goes home and identifies all the tasks that he must complete in an eight-hour shift. Based on the nurse manager's description of the UAPs experience and skills, he assigns tasks to himself and to them. Finally, Jon develops a written mini-job description for himself and the UAPs. The next day he asks the nurse manager to review the job descriptions he has developed and asks for input. She is thrilled with the job descriptions and feels they are very appropriate. He then asks her to provide at least two hours of scheduled time for his team to get to know each other and to establish some guidelines and Jon also requests one eight-hour shift when he and the two nurse's aides can have half of a normal assignment to try the new job descriptions, work out any bugs, and become comfortable with each others' expectations.

Case Study Questions

1. Is Jon using an appropriate delegation process to solve an immediate problem?
2. What are the advantages and disadvantages of the plan Jon has described?
3. What factors should Jon consider when he determines what is appropriate for delegation?

LEARNING RESOURCES

Discussion Questions

1. What are some advantages and disadvantages of delegation?
2. What legal and ethical considerations do nurses who delegate tasks need to consider?
3. When a task is delegated, who then has the authority, responsibility, and accountability for the task?
4. Can all UAPs perform the same tasks? Provide a rationale for your answer.
5. Are there any tasks that managers should not delegate to their subordinates? If so, what are they, and why should they not be delegated?

Study Questions

Matching: Write the correct response in front of each term.

J	1. Delegator	A.	to generate new solutions to problems
I	2. Delegate		
H	3. Supervision	B.	failure to act in accordance with established standards
G	4. Nursing activities		
F	5. Nonnursing activities		
B	6. Negligence	C.	a source useful in exploring ethical problems
D	7. Nurse practice act		
E	8. Board of nursing	D.	a set of rules that governs nursing practice
C	9. ANA's Code for Nurses		
A	10. Adaptors	E.	to function to interpret and enforce the law

F. tasks necessary to support client care

G. tasks necessary to provide care to clients

H. guidance to accomplish a specific task or activity

I. the individual who accepts a new task

J. the individual who assigns a task to another

SUPPLEMENTAL READINGS

Barter, M. & Furmidge, M.L. (1994). Unlicensed assistive personnel: Issues relating to delegation and supervision. *Journal of Nursing Administration,* 24(4), 36-40.

Nagelkerk, J. & Henry, B. (1992-1993). Power delegating. *Graduating Nurse,* 56-57.

Chapter 16

Nursing Care Delivery Systems

STUDY FOCUS

Nursing care modality or the nursing care delivery system of the organization is important in the allocation of resources and in the control of decision making about client care. The type of care modality determines, to a large extent, whether professional practice exists. Nursing care delivery systems are a mechanism to organize and deliver care to clients. The four basic elements of nursing care delivery systems that individuals consider when designing systems are clinical decision making, work allocation, communication, and management. The practice model links the mission statement, professionals, and clients in the delivery of care.

Selecting or designing a nursing care delivery system is a major task and requires a series of strategic decisions. The four strategic decisions needed include developing a philosophy of resource use, choosing a delivery system, developing practice expectations, and designing the role of the registered nurse. The six types of care modalities are functional, private duty, team, primary, case management, and the current evolving care delivery types. Four of these — functional, team, primary, and case management — have been used in hospitals.

Private duty nursing, the oldest type of care modality, is a model in which the nurse cares for one client. This model is very positive for both the nurse and client and fosters a close relationship; however, it is very costly, and job security is low. Group nursing originated from private duty and was an attempt to decrease costs by grouping clients in a hospital ward. The clients then paid the nurse directly. Total client care also originated from private duty nursing as a method of providing total care for a group of clients during one shift.

Functional nursing is the assignment of tasks to personnel prepared for that function. Examples of task assignments include medication administration, intravenous administration, baths, and vital signs. Functional nursing is efficient, but client and nurse satisfaction is low. Team nursing involves the coordination of care by a registered nurse (RN) who assigns work to RNs, LPNs and nurse's aides. The assigned team members provide the majority of care to their assigned clients. Team nursing is cost effective, and each member's skills are used. Modular nursing evolved from team nursing and clusters clients geographically with a group approach to care.

Primary nursing is the first professional practice model and designates 24-hour accountability for assigned clients from admission to discharge. The RN coordinates care and is accountable for the outcomes. The advantages to primary care include close client-nurse relationships and holistic care. However, the cost of care increases with the attention of a professional staff. Case management is the coordination, monitoring, and procuring of services for the multiple needs of clients. Case management may occur only in the hospital, based on populations, or across the healthcare cycle of the individual. Its advantages include cost-effectiveness through a holistic approach to care. Managed care originated from case management and is focused on specific client types and outcomes. Critical paths are one method to manage the care and resources of clients through a written plan that identifies key activities and treatments necessary at prescribed time frames. The current evolving types of care delivery systems are mixed client care models. They are the second generation of professional practice models in nursing. The new evolving types tend to focus on costs, quality, and professional practice.

Managers and clinical nurses are challenged to design client care delivery systems that are cost-effective, provide quality care, and ensure client satisfaction. Important factors nurses must consider when designing care modalities are the staff, assignments, nursing and physician diagnoses, the reporting structure, decision-making autonomy, communication channels, and cost. Political, economic, and social forces are pressuring nurses to treat healthcare as a business with identifiable outcomes and client satisfaction. Nurses are challenged to restructure or design nursing care delivery systems to provide holistic, cost-effective client care.

LEARNING TOOLS

Group Activity: Understanding Nursing Care Delivery Systems

Purpose: To critically examine your philosophy of nursing and apply it to the design of a nursing care delivery system. This exercise entails designing a professional nursing care delivery system that you feel will provide top quality, cost effective care to satisfied consumers by workers who enjoy their work.

Directions: First determine the four strategic decisions about resource use, delivery systems, practice expectations, and the role of the RN. Questions that will help guide your decision making:

a. What is your philosophy of resource use? Should all clients have equal access to all types of equipment, procedures, medications, supplies? Who should determine what is to be ordered for each unit and in what quantities? Should all nurses and unlicensed assistive personnel (UAP) have access to all supplies and resources? How will manpower be distributed?

b. What existing nursing care delivery system will you use? Or will you design or restructure an existing care delivery system to better meet the needs of your client population and organization?

c. What are the practice expectations for each level of care provider? What are the practice expectations for the management team? Will you have working managers? How does nursing interface with other healthcare professionals in your organization? Will your nursing care delivery system foster collaboration and consultation in a multidisciplinary team approach?

d. What is the role of the RN? Will the RN be responsible for supervision, coordination, and provision of care? What will the roles of the other healthcare providers be? Who will delegate work and what process will be used?

Now examine the key components of practice when designing your nursing care delivery system:

a. Composition and skill mix of your staff — What skills are needed to accomplish client care activities? How will the staff be assigned to accomplish the work?

b. Nursing and physician diagnoses — What are the common medical and nursing diagnoses for your client population? How can the diagnostic needs of clients best be met?

c. Reporting procedures — How will reports be given from one shift to another? What type of report will be used? How will physicians be notified of client changes?

d. Communication channels — How will nurses, clients, physicians, and other healthcare workers communicate needs and changes in procedures? How will the manager communicate with all healthcare members? Will the communication network be written or verbal?

e. Cost-effectiveness — How will supplies and equipment be used? What mechanisms will be in place to encourage cost-effective care? Will critical pathways be used?

After you have thought about all these questions, design a nursing care delivery system by either modifying an existing one or constructing your own. This exercise will help you determine what type of care delivery structure you prefer, give you ideas to share in your work environment, and force you to analyze the use of precious resources.

CASE STUDY

Mary Jo is the nurse manager of the respiratory unit in Middlesville, North Carolina. Middlesville hospital has been experiencing budgetary problems, and Mary Jo has been instructed to cut costs in manpower. Mary Jo designs a new care delivery system. She informs the staff the next morning that the unit will fill all of the empty positions with UAPs. She has made the assignments as follows: two RNs are assigned to pass medications and intravenous fluids, two LPNs are assigned to give baths, another LPN is assigned to do treatments, and one UAP is assigned vital signs, meal preparation, and transportation duties. Two RNs are floated to intensive care to work.

Case Study Questions

1. What type of care modality did Mary Jo design?
2. What are the advantages and disadvantages of this type of care delivery system?
3. What factors did Mary Jo need to consider?

LEARNING RESOURCES

Discussion Questions

1. What are the advantages and disadvantages of each of the six types of nursing care delivery?
2. What are the four common types of nursing care delivery systems used in hospitals?
3. What factors should nurses consider when designing or restructuring a care delivery system?
4. What social, political, and economic factors influence the delivery of client care? How?
5. What is the clinical nurse's role in designing care delivery systems?

Study Questions

Matching: Write the letter of the correct response in front of each term.

J   1. Nursing care modality

I   2. Private duty nursing

E   3. Team nursing

D   4. Primary nursing

C   5. Managed care

B   6. Case management

F   7. Functional nursing

A   8. Current evolving type

H   9. Total client care

G   10. Group nursing

A. a mixed model approach to provide care

B. care provided based on specific types of clients and resource use

C. the coordination of care to meet the multiple needs of clients

D. the assignment of clients to one nurse who has 24-hour accountability

E. coordination of care with RN, LPN, and aide assignments by an RN to a group of clients

F. the assignment of tasks to either RNs, LPNs, or aides

G. when nurses provide care to one or more clients for one shift

H. when clients are grouped together and cared for by one nurse

I. when one nurse provides care to one client

J. a method of organizing and delivering care to clients

SUPPLEMENTAL READINGS

Gollard, L. & Soo Hoo, W. (1993). Maximizing limited resources through TEAMCARE. *Nursing Management,* 24(11), 36-38, & 40-43.

Wolf, G., Boland, S. & Aukerman, M. (1994). A transformational model for the practice of professional nursing: Part I, the model. *Journal of Nursing Administration,* 24(4), 51-57.

Chapter 17

Case Management and Managed Care

STUDY FOCUS

The complexity and demands of cost, quality, and access create the need for nurses to design innovative care delivery systems. Managed care and case management are two innovative methods for organizing and providing services to clients. Managed care is the broader concept from which case management is one method of approaching client care to achieve cost, quality, and access. Managed care is organizing and sequencing caregiving at the client-provider level to achieve cost and quality objectives. Health maintenance organizations, privately managed indemnity health insurance plans, and preferred provider organizations are the most commonly associated structures related to managed care. These organizations emphasize lowered costs with maximum value.

Case management, on the other hand, is a system of assessing, planning, procuring services, and delivering care to meet the multiple needs of clients. Case management links services with the care needs of clients to maximize outcomes. Case management is commonly used in hospitals. It can be used with a population focus or over a health cycle of an individual. Four basic principles of case management are coordination of holistic care, health promotion through risk and transition, disciplined resource use, and follow-up care through episodes and settings. Case management infers accompaniment, a professional client-nurse relationship, focused on holistic care to prevent fragmentation and to ensure continuity and the coordination of services.

In many instances, case management is used for high priority clients to decrease costs and improve quality of care. Priority clients include those who exhibit recidivism and frequent emergency use, unpredictable care needs, complications, co-morbidities or variances, high risk profiles, and costly care. Development of a case management program entails the following step-by-step process: assessing the population and organizational needs; identifying high-volume or high-risk cases; determining goals; forming a multidisciplinary team; designing a critical pathway; conducting a pilot project; and evaluating.

Critical pathways are used in both case management and managed care and consist of key incidents, treatments, and events that are associated with improved outcomes. Critical pathways are usually developed by multidisciplinary teams based on professional standards and illustrated in a decision tree format. Standards of care are formalized through a written critical pathway, and variances in client progress can be detected immediately and corrected.

Healthcare demands require nurses to expand their care coordination role and decrease their care provision role in many of the new care modalities. In case management and managed care, nurses play pivotal roles in coordinating client care and leading multidisciplinary teams. Clinical nurses are now clinical managers of care for either individual clients, groups of clients, or teams of clients. Managers who are selecting care modalities should examine the new models in relationship to the integration of nursing care, continuity of assignments, and coordination, organization, and delivery of care. Nurses are in a unique position to increase their level of responsibility, authority, and accountability. Are nurses ready to take a major leadership role in the organization, coordination, and delivery of client care?

LEARNING TOOLS

Group Activity: Understanding Critical Pathways

Purpose: To explore the role and design of critical pathways in the delivery of healthcare to clients.

Directions: Divide yourselves into small groups of four. Each small group should discuss the role of critical pathways in healthcare delivery, determining what types of client problems/diagnoses lend themselves to critical pathway development. Select one client problem/diagnosis and sketch out a critical pathway. (Each small group should bring a critical pathway from where they work [clinic, hospital] and share it with everyone during the study session.)

When each small group shares its critical pathway, compare your critical pathway with those that the hospitals or clinics where you practice use. Notice the critical steps or client points at which treatment, medical, nursing, or other healthcare worker intervention is required. Also note the length of time for each and the desired client outcomes. Finally, note the similarities and differences in the structure of the critical pathways among the various groups, hospitals, and clinics. Discuss and summarize these key points.

CASE STUDY

Bob is a family nurse practitioner who works for a health maintenance organization (HMO) in Orlando, Florida. Bob is responsible for coordinating the care for a case load of clients who enroll in the HMO. Bob's boss has told him that the objectives of his care coordination and delivery should focus on lowering costs with maximum value and quality outcomes. Bob is careful to refer clients to only those specialists listed on the preferred provider list since he knows that they have agreed to a discounted payment arrangement. Bob also provides holistic care with an emphasis on health promotion and wellness.

Case Study Questions

1. What type of care modality is Bob using at the HMO? Is it case management or managed care?
2. What are the characteristics of case management versus managed care?
3. Can Bob refer outside of the preferred provider specialist list that the HMO provides for him?

LEARNING RESOURCES

Discussion Questions

1. What was the impetus for the design of case management and managed care?
2. What are the differences and similarities of case management and managed care, and in what types of situations would you use each of these care modalities?
3. What are critical pathways? Why are critical pathways important in cost containment and improved quality?

4. What are the leadership and management challenges for nurses for designing care delivery systems in the future?
5. What is the clinical nurse's role in the provision of care, coordination of care, and the design of new care delivery systems?

Study Questions

True and False: Circle the correct answer.

T	F	1.	Nurses must document their effects upon client outcomes to demonstrate that they can provide cost-effective services.
T	F	2.	Case management is frequently associated with health maintenance organizations and preferred provider organizations.
T	F	3.	Managed care is care coordination and delivery at the provider-client level.
T	F	4.	Managed care typically is used for only high priority clients.
T	F	5.	Critical pathways are used only with case management.
T	F	6.	Case management is a broader term defined as a system of providing structure and focus for client care.
T	F	7.	Mulitdisciplinary teams are essential in a complex healthcare environment.
T	F	8.	Case management entails providing holistic care, the conservation of resources, and care across episodes and settings.
T	F	9.	Case management focuses on continuity of the plan.
T	F	10.	Registered nurses are moving from a care providing role to a care coordinating role.

SUPPLEMENTAL READINGS

Buerhaus, P. (1994). Economics of managed competition and consequences to nurses, Part II. *Nursing Economics, 12*(2), 75-106.

Rheaume, A., Frisch, S., Smith, A., & Kennedy, C. (1994). Case management and nursing practice. *Journal of Nursing Administration, 24*(3), 30-36.

Chapter 18

Communication

STUDY FOCUS

Communication is an essential element in organizing, coordinating, and directing the care of clients. Nurse managers are challenged to create clear communication pathways to facilitate task accomplishment in organizations. Communication is the ability to transmit information to another clearly. Organizational communication is the ability of an agency to transmit information to and from its members expediently and expeditiously. Verbal communication is verbal or written information, and nonverbal communication is transmitted through behaviors. The four distinctions in communication are those between the formal/informal, vertical/horizontal, personal/impersonal, and instrumental/expressive types. Formal communication is the official information sent by designated officials in an agency, and informal is information passed via the grapevine. Vertical communication is boss to employee, and horizontal is peer to peer. Personal communication is when mutual influence occurs, and impersonal is one-sided communication. Instrumental communication is transmitting data essential to complete work, and expressive is data that is tangential to the work that is done.

Communication is both an art and a skill in which a sender and a receiver engage in the transmission of ideas or information. Following are steps in communication whereby information is exchanged: message formation where the sender formulates ideas; message encoding where the sender formulates the idea into verbal or nonverbal components; message transmission where the sender imparts the message; message reception where the receiver in some way acquires the transmission; and message decoding where the receiver interprets the data. In communication, there is always the potential for barriers due to the perception and filtration of information by both the sender and receiver. People have their own unique world view which colors or changes the message to fit their model of the world. Therefore, it is extremely important to keep messages clear, simple, and relevant to the receiver.

Group communication is even more complex than individual communication because of the number of individuals involved. Five common communication networks are used: the wheel, the chain, the Y, the all-channel, and the circle. In centralized organizations, the wheel, the Y, and the chain are used. In democratic organizations the circle and the all-channel networks are used most often.

Communication effectiveness is influenced by the message, the way it is delivered, and the method used to communicate. People tend to respond more positively when they are contacted individually. Discrimination or exclusion raises sensitivities and distracts from the message. It is important to determine if the message is understood by the receiver. Feedback is an important managerial tool and enhances subordinates' performance. Clear, immediate, honest input is required for effective outcomes.

Because they work in complex, technologically advanced environments with people who are not well, nurses have typically been targets of criticism from clients, physicians, and other healthcare workers. Strategies for dealing with critical individuals include agreeing with the criticism, seeking further information, and guiding the criticism toward problem solving. At times, managers must use constructive criticism in order to improve subordinates' poor performance. In these cases, blame should not be the focus; instead the focus should be on analysis of the problems and a formulation of goals to be achieved in order to solve them. Constructive feedback should be given in an appropriate environment and time. Specific behavioral statements should be used to describe the poor behavior.

Nurses must also remember that image is important in communicating professionalism to the public. Dress and appearance reflect heavily upon the public's perception of the nurse's image. Language can be used by nurses to clearly articulate their values and the nature of their work with clients.

Multicultural diversity, another current concern, is reflected in ethnic, cultural, and linguistic diversity. Managers must be aware of methods to facilitate cultural diversity in the work environment. Cultural diversity in nursing education has been facilitated by recruiting people of color, providing preceptor programs, personalizing recruitment, formalizing nontraditional admission criteria, establishing a culturally sensitive learning environment, and recruiting faculty of color.

LEARNING TOOLS

Group Activity: Exploring Verbal and Nonverbal Communication

Purpose: To identify the impact of verbal and nonverbal communication when interacting with others. In light of the fact that approximately 55% of a speaker's message is the result of facial and body language (the majority is facial); 38% the vocal quality; and only 7% the actual words used, this activity is designed to help you assess your communication style with others.

Directions: Divide yourselves into groups of three. One person will be sending a message; one person will be receiving the message; and one person will observe the interaction and then provide feedback. First, have one person describe the most important thing that has happened to him or her within the past year. Three minutes should be allowed for the interaction. Then reverse the procedure until everyone has had an opportunity to observe, send, and receive a message. Observers should jot down comments about verbal and nonverbal communication. The following observer checklist may be used. Secondly, have each person describe the worst thing that has happened to him or her in the last year. Again, use the observer checklist to record comments.

Afterwards, everyone should share his or her observer comments with the group. Talk with each other about the impact verbal and nonverbal communication has upon the content of the message. Receivers should discuss the verbal or nonverbal activity that they focused on the most. Discuss how mannerisms or nonverbal behaviors can distract or support a message.

Observer Checklist

For each of the categories, prompts are provided. Write down the major and minor verbal and nonverbal characteristics that you noted for both the sender and receiver.

Facial Expression

1. Note the eyes and mouth for expressiveness—is the sender relating happiness? sadness?

2. How is the receiver responding?

Sender   Receiver

Body Language

1. Note the arms, hands, legs, shoulders, and hips. How is the sender illustrating his or her message?
2. How is the receiver acknowledging the message?
3. Is the sender's message supportive, disinterested, or boring?
4. What impact is the sender's message having upon the receiver? Is the sender changing the content of the message based upon the receiver's feedback?

Sender   Receiver

Vocal Quality

1. Is the tone, pitch, and volume consistent with the message?
2. Is the sender's message spoken in a monotone? Is there variation in tone to make an impact upon the receiver?
3. Is the sender forceful? weak? bored? interested? animated? eager?
4. Does the sender use a strong, soft, reflective, or humorous presentation?

Sender   Receiver

Articulated Words

1. What actual verbal message was sent?
2. What words were used to send the message?
3. Were metaphors used? Were red flags or emotionally charged words used?

Sender   Receiver

CASE STUDY

Martha is the nurse manager of an operating room in Lake Worth, Florida. Jill is a registered nurse who has worked in the operating room for three years. Lately, Jill has been having problems completing the documentation that she is required to do, has been taking long breaks, and is refusing to scrub for several physicians. Martha is informed that staffing is short and that they will need her to cover cases just to get through the day. Martha enjoys scrubbing and is very willing to help out to facilitate a smooth progression of clients through the operating room. After Martha has finished her second case, the charge nurse informs her that they are one case behind. Martha asks if there was an emergency or a late case. The charge nurse says no, but that Jill took a 45-minute break and refused to scrub for a physician. Martha walks into the conference room where Jill is reading a book. Martha angrily reprimands Jill in front of two staff members and tells Jill to either scrub for the physician or go home.

Case Study Questions

1. Did Martha respond in an appropriate fashion?
2. What other strategies could Martha have used to manage this situation?
3. What are characteristics of constructive feedback?

LEARNING RESOURCES

Discussion Questions

1. What is essential for effective communication to occur?
2. What types of communication networks are there? What types of communication networks are used in decentralized and centralized organizations?
3. What are effective methods to facilitate cultural diversity within the work environment?
4. What are the steps in information exchange?
5. Why are nurses targeted for criticism? What strategies can nurses use to handle criticism?

Study Questions

True and False: Circle the correct answer.

T F 1. Verbal communication includes both affective and expressive behaviors.

T F 2. Positive communication techniques include agreeing uncritically and reassuringly.

T F 3. Individual communication is more complex than group communication because it is so intensive.

T F 4. Horizontally decentralized organizations are more efficient than centralized organizations.

T F 5. Feedback should be used carefully and only when absolutely necessary since it inhibits effective communication.

T F 6. To respond effectively to communication, place blame on others.

T F 7. The major part of any communication is the words we say to others.

T F 8. Effective communication is clear, direct, and straightforward.

T F 9. Metaphors and political language can be used by nurse leaders to influence governmental officials.

T F 10. Nurses are often targets of verbal abuse.

SUPPLEMENTAL READINGS

Goldberg, M.C. (1994). A new imperative for listening to clients. *Journal of Nursing Administration, 24*(3), 11-12.

Martin, K., Wimberley, D., & O'Keefe, K. (1994). Resolving conflict in a multicultural nursing department. *Nursing Management, 25*(1), 49-51.

Chapter 19

Motivation

STUDY FOCUS

Motivation is a complex process requiring strong leadership and management skills to creatively enhance employee productivity. Nurse managers of healthcare organizations are faced with trying to increase employee productivity while maintaining or decreasing labor costs. Motivation is the perception of the person toward a goal which energizes them to act. An activity is the basic unit of behavior. Individuals perform activities based on their motives or needs, what they desire or want. Nurse managers are challenged to motivate employees to work in a way that achieves organizational goals expeditiously. Energizing, facilitating, and maintaining high levels of employee productivity is often problematic.

Traditionally, managers of bureaucratic organizations use direct supervision to control employees; whereas managers using a human relations approach in decentralized organizations employ the methods of participation and cooperation. Many motivational models have been developed to help guide managers in motivating employees to maximum productivity. The needs satisfaction model states that there is a felt need followed by an activity or behavioral response. Then a process results to decrease frustration and meet individual needs. Individual needs arise from both internal and external motivating forces. Internal motivation is a personal desire to achieve and accomplish. On the other hand, external motivation is a stimulus external to an individual which generates an incentive to complete an activity.

Maslow's hierarchy of needs theory is based on levels of human needs starting with basic needs and ending with self-actualization. Maslow's hierarchy includes five levels — physiological drives, safety and security needs, belonging needs, esteem and ego needs, and self-actualization. Maslow's work was refined by Alderfer who collapsed the five levels to three which include existence, relatedness, and growth needs.

Herzberg's motivation-hygiene theory describes two categories of needs, hygiene or maintenance factors and motivators. Hygiene or maintenance factors are security, status, money, working conditions, inter-personal relations, supervision, and policies and administration. Motivators include the need for growth and development, advancement, increased responsibility, challenging work, recognition, and achievement. Motivators encourage superior performance while hygiene factors maintain satisfaction.

McClelland's theory describes three basic needs: achievement, power, and affiliation. McClelland's theory lends itself to self-assessment. Nursing leaders were found to have no need to moderately high levels of need for power, low levels of affiliation needs, high levels of self-control needs, and minimal achievement motivation.

Expectancy theories, including Vroom's, examine the attractiveness of an outcome, a valence, and the likelihood that the outcome will occur. In these theories, employees assess the value of an outcome and the degree to which individuals perceive that they can attain the reward. Then they decide whether they will expend the energy to perform the activity.

Job characteristics theory examines the job, the individual, and the outcome. Core job dimensions of the theory include task identity, task significance, skill variety, and autonomy and feedback. The core job dimensions interact with three critical psychological states — the meaningfulness of the work, responsibility for outcomes, and the actual result of the work. The outcomes may improve productivity, enhance quality, decrease turnover and absenteeism, and improve personal and professional job satisfaction.

McGregor published theory X and theory Y. Theory X's basic assumptions are that employees are lazy and nonproductive and require close supervision. It portrays employees as resistant to autonomy and unable to assume responsibility. In contrast, theory Y's basic assumptions are that employees enjoy autonomy and need only guidance as opposed to supervision. Employees are depicted as creative, self-directed individuals who embrace responsibility and autonomy.

The classic Hawthorne studies were conducted in 1924 at the Hawthorne plant of Western Electric. The studies examined the motivation and productivity of assembly line workers. Several variables — including improving lighting, scheduling breaks, providing lunches, and shortening work hours — were studied with control and experimental groups. To the researchers' surprise, all the variables had a significant positive impact upon employee productivity. Even after all the variables were withdrawn productivity climbed. Study outcomes showed that interpersonal relationships were also a significant factor in motivating employees.

Nurses are motivated by personal, professional, and economic recognition. Verbal feedback has been identified as the most meaningful form of recognition for nurses. Five types of recognition are verbal feedback, written feedback, public acknowledgment, advancement and growth opportunities, and compensation. Other major influences motivating nurses are job enjoyment, quality care, caring by their superior/boss, adequate staffing, and a safe work environment. Nurses are compensated economically via base, variable, and indirect pay. Base pay is salary for work performed; variable pay includes bonuses and incentive pay, while indirect pay includes benefits such as health insurance, sick time, and vacation pay. Many employees view pay as an entitlement. It does not motivate them, but it does prevents dissatisfaction when adequate.

Managers must structure environments to enhance productivity. Elements that affect motivation include goals, expectations, feedback, reinforcement, responsibility, trust, and rewards. Motivating techniques include using formal rewards, tailoring rewards to the employee, and providing immediate feedback. The current trends in nursing are to use formal recognition by designating heroes and heroines and reframing responsibilities.

LEARNING TOOLS

Role Play

Motivating Subordinates to Improve Productivity

Character One = Jo Ellen is the nurse manager of a neurorespiratory unit of a medium-sized hospital in Beaumont, Texas. Jo Ellen believes in rewarding staff for superior performance and tailors reward based on individual accomplishments.

Character Two = Bob is an RN who was hired ten years ago and has been doing an adequate, but not exemplary job.

Character Three = Jon is an RN who was hired five years ago and who consistently exhibits superior performance in client care.

Character Four = Jane is an RN who was hired one year ago and consistently performs well.

Jo Ellen is preparing annual reviews (performance appraisals) on all of her employees. She knows that Jon, Bob, and Jane are best friends and share information with each other. Jo Ellen wants to reward Jon and Jane for their exemplary performance, but does not want Bob disgruntled. Jo Ellen decides to give special merit pay to Jon and award him the neurological nurse of the year because he consistently performs outstandingly. Jo Ellen also puts Jane's name in for the hospital's professional nurse of the year award and sends her to a national neurosurgical nursing convention in California. One morning, Jo Ellen enters the neurorespiratory unit to see Jane, Bob, and Jon arguing loudly in the conference room. Upon entering the conference room, Bob aggressively approaches Jo Ellen and demands an explanation for her poor choices as a manager. Bob demands to know why his ten years of loyal service were not recognized. What should Jo Ellen do?

Role-play Questions:

1. What should Jo Ellen say? Should she give Bob a reward?
2. What strategies can be used to motivate Bob to work harder?
3. How can Jo Ellen manage the situation to empower all three individuals?

Role-play Worksheet

CHARACTERS	STUDENT ASSIGNED
Jo Ellen, the nurse manager	_____
Bob, RN of 10 years	_____
Jon, RN of 5 years	_____
Jane, RN of 1 year	_____

Which character have you been assigned?

What are your character's goals in this situation?

How can the other characters assist you in achieving your goals?

What might the other characters do to hinder you in achieving your goals?

What strategies and probes do you plan to use in this situation?

CASE STUDY

Jackie is a charge nurse on the 11–7 shift at Middleville Hospital in Little Rock, Arkansas. Jackie's leadership style includes directing employees to accomplish tasks. She feels that the nurse's aides, licensed practical nurses (LPN), and orderlies are lazy and do only what they are required to do. Jackie requires them to report to her any client changes, large or small, because she feels they cannot handle responsibility. Jackie has developed detailed, step-by-step procedures for her staff to follow to prevent mistakes.

Case Study Questions

1. What motivational theory is Jackie practicing from?
2. What are the characteristics of this theory?
3. Is this an effective theory to practice leadership behaviors?

LEARNING RESOURCES

Discussion Questions

1. What types of rewards motivate nurses to improve productivity?
2. What did the Hawthorne studies show? Why were the Hawthorne studies' results important to managers?
3. What is the difference between internal and external motivation? How can a nurse manager capitalize on these?
4. What is the difference between the needs satisfaction model and Vroom's theory?
5. How can you apply Maslow's hierarchy of needs theory to nursing management?

Study Questions

Matching: Write the letter of the corret response in front of each term.

G 1. Motivation
H 2. Motives
I 3. External motivation
D 4. Variable pay
A 5. Activity
J 6. Internal motivation
B 7. Indirect pay
C 8. Base pay
F 9. Vroom's theory
E 10. McClelland's theory

A. a unit of human behavior
B. benefits like sick and vacation time
C. salary received for work completed
D. gain sharing, bonuses, and incentive pay
E. identifies the basic needs people possess
F. represents valence, instrumentality, and expectancy
G. energizing and eliciting human activity
H. wants, desires, and drives
I. individuals who provide incentives for activity
J. accomplishments arising from within the individual

SUPPLEMENTAL READING

Kelley, R. & Caplan, J. (1993). How Bell Labs creates star performers. *Harvard Business Review, 71*(4), 128-139.
Keyes, M. (1994). Recognition and reward: A unit-based program. *Nursing Management, 25*(2), 52-54.

Chapter 20 ●
Power

STUDY FOCUS

Power gives us control and freedom. Power is the ability to influence another's actions in order to attain a scarce resource. Empowerment is giving responsibility and accountability to individuals to complete tasks. There is personal and professional power. Personal power is the extent to which individuals can influence events through their own personal effort, while professional power is influence which results from doing a good job and interacting with colleagues.

The eight mechanisms people use to gain power include assertiveness, ingratiation, rationality, sanctions, exchange, upward appeal, blocking, and coalitions. Assertiveness is standing up for your rights without infringing on others' rights. Ingratiation is praising someone for a job well done in hopes of gaining recognition for your support. Rationality is the logical presentation of ideas. Sanctions include the use of threats and negative activities to gain a desired response. Exchanges are trades for services or goods in which both parties receive something desired. Upward appeals involve the act of seeking opinion of a higher authority about a decision. Blocking is stopping someone's activities or progress by threatening them, ignoring them, or physically interfering with their progress. Coalitions are the banding together of individuals for the purpose of a single voice.

Raven and French identify five sources of power. Reward power is the use of praise, pay, promotions, or advancements. Coercive power is the use of force such as threatening to fire an individual or to discipline them. Expert power is based on knowledge, competence, and skill. Referent power is based on a person's interpersonal appeal, charisma, and image. Legitimate power is based on the job title or position a person holds. Other sources of power include connection, a network of powerful people or information sources, and informational power, the control of special information.

In organizations, formal power is attained through position. Nurse managers must use power to be effective in leading the staff in care delivery. The four sources of organizational power include structural position, personal characteristics, expertise, and opportunity. Structural position is positional power and includes centrality, control of uncertainty, and control over resources. Individuals accrue power by the centrality of their work to the organization's mission and the visibility and discretion associated with their job. Personal characteristics incorporate the culture, values, and mix.

To be powerful, one must be able to access support, information, and resources, and must be aware of opportunities, in order to seize advancement or achievements. Those who use power positively resolve conflicts with creativity, innovation, and novelty; whereas, those who use power ineffectively create barriers, decrease efficiency, and encourage distrust and uncomfortable work environments. Strategies to gain and maintain power include gaining access to information, controlling resources, accessing key decision makers, and networking with powerful individuals.

Power moments refer to those occasions when one individual interferes with another's power. Strategies that may be used during power moments include fights, which engage two or more people in a struggle for the same resource; negotiation, where two or more people respectfully discuss the situation and come to an agreement; and collaboration, where two or more individuals cooperate to determine a solution. Multiple power sources need to be used to avoid diminished power resources. Political strategies include forming coalitions, bargaining, lobbying, posturing or bluffing, and increasing visibility. Empowering others promotes excellence and motivates others.

LEARNING TOOLS
Self-assessment

Power Inventory

Introduction: Power is an important aspect of our personal and professional lives. Understanding your own level of comfort with power will help you gain support and resources in your work environment.

Directions: 1. Write a brief response to the statement under each item. 2. Circle a number on the continuum that best corresponds with how you view yourself.

(1 = Strongly Agree, 2 = Moderately Agree, 3 = Agree, 4 = Somewhat Agree, 5 = Disagree)

1. I am sensitive to where power exists in organizations.   1 2 3 4 5

_____

_____

_____

2. I feel that power can be used effectively without disadvantaging individuals.   1 2 3 4 5

_____

_____

_____

3. I feel comfortable taking risks.   1 2 3 4 5

_____

_____

_____

4. I try to obtain additional resources in my work setting.   1 2 3 4 5

_____

_____

_____

5. I engage in activities to strengthen my power base.   1 2 3 4 5

_____

_____

_____

6. I avoid activities that will decrease my power.   1 2 3 4 5

_____

_____

_____

7. I feel I have a base of colleagues whom I can count on to support my ideas or projects.   1 2 3 4 5

_____

_____

_____

8. I enjoy taking charge of situations or projects to accomplish goals.   1 2 3 4 5

_____

_____

_____

9. I enjoy speaking in front of groups, meeting new people, and being the center of attention.   1 2 3 4 5

_____

_____

_____

10. I enjoy competing for resources with others.   1 2 3 4 5

_____

_____

_____

Scoring: Review the scoring of each of the 10 questions. Count the number of items that you ranked high (3, 4, or 5). Were the majority of your rankings high? Examine the items that you scored high. If you scored many items high you probably do not feel comfortable gaining and using power. Focus on one or two items where you would like to gain confidence in gaining power. Identify activities that you can engage in to empower yourself in personal and professional interactions.

CASE STUDY

Sandy, a staff nurse on a 66-bed medical-surgical unit in Sagers, Hawaii, decides to establish a strong power base for herself. She has read a book about power mechanisms and decides to experiment with them. Sandy arrives on the unit and notices that her assignment is heavy. She decides to address the charge nurse by stating the facts about the number of clients she has, and their acuity levels. She requests that the assignment be adjusted in light of the data presented. The charge nurse refuses Sandy's request and walks away. Sandy decides to approach the nurse manager and again presents all the facts. The nurse manager intervenes and modifies the assignment. Sandy meets Ruth Ann, a clinical nurse specialist, in the hall and praises her for the new client care delivery model she developed. Finally, Sandy begins care delivery and realizes she cannot handle the turning and positioning alone. She seeks assistance from Judy and says she will return the favor. Judy agrees to help.

Case Study Questions

1. What power mechanisms did Sandy use?
2. Is Sandy empowering herself by using these power mechanisms?
3. What else can Sandy do to garner power?

LEARNING RESOURCES

Discussion Questions

1. What are the five power bases described by French and Raven?
2. What is the difference between personal power-oriented individuals and institutionalized power-oriented individuals?
3. How can a nurse manager empower the staff? What effect does empowerment have on care delivery?
4. What are effective strategies for staff nurses to use to empower themselves and their colleagues?
5. What are the differences between fight, negotiation, and collaboration? Identify a situation in which each might be appropriate.

Study Questions

Matching: Write the correct letter of the correct response in front of each term.

D	1. Power	A. power based on charisma and interpersonal appeal
C	2. Empowerment	B. the authority to act based on position
J	3. Reward power	C. providing the opportunity for others to take responsibility and accountability for their work
H	4. Coercive power	D. influencing an individual or group in order to gain a scarce resource
I	5. Expert power	E. lavishing praise on another in order to gain favor
A	6. Referent power	F. formation of a group for the purpose of a single voice in order to affect change
B	7. Legitimate power	G. taking a concern to a higher authority
E	8. Ingratiation	H. the use of threats, discipline, or negative consequences
G	9. Upward appeal	I. individuals who possess special skills or talents
F	10. Coalitions	J. providing a pay raise, promotion, or advancement

SUPPLEMENTAL READINGS

Kippenbrock, T.A. (1992). Power at meetings: Strategies to move people. *Nursing Economics, 10*(4), 282-286.
Tebbitt, B.V. (1993). Demystifying organizational empowerment. *Journal of Nursing Administration, 23*(1), 18-23.

STUDY FOCUS

Conflict is natural and can be a useful growth experience for individuals. Conflict arises between two or more individuals from a perceived threat to their wants, needs, feelings, behaviors, or attitudes. Organizational conflict arises from competition for the limited available resources in an organization. Job conflict is the struggle between individual and organizational goals. Conflict occurs because of discord between one individual's values, philosophies, and beliefs and those of other individuals. When conflict is handled positively, there can be personal or professional growth; improved relationships; and increased productivity, creativity, and satisfaction. When it is handled poorly, fear, retaliation, anger, and hostility are the result.

Conflict can be categorized three ways — intrapersonal, interpersonal, and intergroup. Intrapersonal conflict arises within an individual from two competing demands or ideas. Interpersonal conflict is the battle between two or more individuals arising from miscommunication or differences in values. Intergroup conflict is the result of struggles between two or more groups. Conflict can be either competitive, when the individuals strive to win, or it may be disruptive, when the intent is to defeat, eliminate, or harm the opponent.

Pondy (1967) has identified five stages of conflict. The first stage is antecedent conditions, which are the conditions that begin stirring the pot of discontent. Examples could include the competition for resources, differing goals, or a lack of individual responsibility. The second stage, perceived conflict, emerges, and emotions become charged. During the third stage, an individual has a felt conflict and expresses these emotions. The individual initiates behavior to correct or alleviate the felt conflict either by negatively talking about the other individuals, by initiating actions to correct the situation, or by removing himself from the uncomfortable environment. Manifest behavior occurs in the fourth stage when the individual acts and either resolves or suppresses the conflict. The fifth and final stage, aftermath to the conflict, occurs when there is an effect, either resolution to the conflict or a cyclic process in which increasing antecedent behaviors take place.

There are three strategies that can be used to resolve organizational conflicts: bargaining; using rules, procedures, and administrative control; and using a system integrator. Nurses can experience conflict in the form of role overload, in which they are required to do the work of other healthcare disciplines; or in role ambiguity, in which the nurses' responsibilities and duties expand without a job description change; or role stress, where a nurse's boss has one idea about her job and the nurse has a different perception.

Effectively managing conflict is essential for positive work groups. There are three frameworks for resolving conflict: defensive, compromise, and creative. The defensive mode leaves individuals feeling both losses and wins. Strategies for defensively addressing conflict are separating the competing parties, suppressing conflict, restricting the conflict, smoothing over the conflict through change, and avoiding the conflict. A compromise mode solves conflict through negotiation until a mutually acceptable solution is reached in which each party receives something and forfeits something. The creative problem-solving mode is the best possible scenario, where all parties gain and do not feel a loss. In creative conflict resolution, a five-step process is used: initiating discussion at a set time in private, understanding and respecting differences, empathizing with each party, engaging in an assertive discussion, and agreeing on a solution.

Conflict resolution techniques include avoiding, withholding, smoothing over, accommodating, forcing, competing, compromising, confronting, collaborating, bargaining, and problem solving. Outcomes for conflict resolution include win-win, win-lose, and lose-lose. Win-lose is when one party wins without concern about the other. Win-win occurs when both parties are satisfied with the outcome, and lose-lose is when neither party gets what they want. Nurse managers are challenged to build positive interdisciplinary work teams, and the process usually requires conflict management and resolution. One group strategy nurses have used to manage conflict is collective bargaining, which is aimed at preventing total control by employers over work conditions, skill mix, and compensation.

LEARNING TOOLS

Self-assessment

Introduction: Conflict management is an important skill for nurses to acquire in order to build teams, to work in complex client care situations, and to obtain scarce resources. By evaluating your conflict management style, you can gain insight into what strategies

have been effective methods for resolving conflict. Diane Huber developed the Perceived Conflict Scale to measure the conflict among hospital nurses.

The Perceived Conflict Scale

Purpose: To become aware of job conflict levels. If you do not work in a healthcare organization, rate the following assessment from the perspective of a student working in the clinical agency.

Directions: Read each question, and circle the number that most accurately represents your feelings. Select option 3 if conflict exists, but you are unable to identify its strength. Each item has a 5-point Likert-type scale: 1 – strongly disagree, 2 – disagree, 3 – neutral, 4 – agree, and 5 – strongly agree.

	Strongly Disagree	Disagree	Neutral	Agree	Strongly Agree
1. Other nurses often disagree with each other about how work on this unit should be handled.	1	2	3	4	5
2. I usually agree with the way other nurses think things should be done on this unit.	1	2	3	4	5
3. My supervisor and I usually agree about what my job is and the requirements I must fulfill.	1	2	3	4	5
4. I usually agree with the decisions my head nurse and supervisor make.	1	2	3	4	5
5. Clients often demand that I do things I simply cannot do.	1	2	3	4	5
6. When I do something that satisfies one person or group, other people are frequently upset with what I have done.	1	2	3	4	5
7. The employees that I see who are from other areas of the hospital are often difficult to deal with.	1	2	3	4	5
8. The various departments that I deal with in the hospital are usually helpful and make it easy for me to do my job.	1	2	3	4	5
9. I frequently encounter problems when I transfer my clients to other units or departments.	1	2	3	4	5
10. Support services (dietary, maintenance, etc.) are readily available when I need them.	1	2	3	4	5
11. Many times, the things that support services are supposed to do are not adequately done, and I either have to argue with another unit or do someone else's job.	1	2	3	4	5
12. I am unable to provide adequate client care because of the time that I spend dealing with hospital rules and red tape.	1	2	3	4	5
13. I often cannot get equipment, supplies, or medications when I need them.	1	2	3	4	5
14. My clients often make requests or need care that I feel I should provide, but cannot because I lack the time or energy.	1	2	3	4	5

15. My obligations to my work frequently conflict with my obligations to family, friends, or myself (outside the job).

16. I often have too many things to do at one time.

Strongly Disagree	Disagree	Neutral	Agree	Strongly Agree
1	2	3	4	5
1	2	3	4	5

Reverse Score Items: For items 2, 3, 4, 8, and 10 reverse the 1-5 Likert scale to score them. For example, if you scored 5, change it to 1; if you scored 1, change it to 5; if you scored 4, change it to 2; and if you scored 2, change it to 4.

Subscales: Name	Items
1. Intrapersonal Conflict	5, 14, 15, 16

*Conflict that arises within the individual from two competing demands.

2. Interpersonal Conflict   1, 2, 3, 4

*Conflict between two or more individuals arising from miscommunication or differences in values.

3. Intergroup/Support Conflict   10, 11, 12, 13

*Conflict between two or more groups that are supportive in work or personal lives. Differences in competition for resources, power, or status may occur.

4. Intergroup/Other Departments   6, 7, 8, 9

*Conflict between two or more groups for resources or services. The conflict may be competitive or disruptive and may center around resources or control.

*Scoring: The higher the mean score, the greater the level of conflict.

Case Study

Jennifer is a nurse manager on a neuroscience unit in Chicago, Illinois. She has been trying to get funding for renovating the neuroscience unit. Jonathan is a nurse manager on the orthopedic unit in the same hospital. The Vice President of Nursing has announced that there is enough money to renovate only one unit in the hospital, and that she would like proposals from both Jennifer and Jonathan because their units are those in the most need for repair. Jennifer calls Jonathan after the meeting and asks if they could meet and discuss the renovation issue. Jonathon eagerly accepts the invitation since he has wanted to work with Jennifer to resolve this conflict of interest.

Jennifer and Jonathan meet with a detailed work plan of desired renovations for each of their units. They both have costs for the projects. Jennifer and Jonathan both agree that they do not want to compete for the renovation because morale will suffer greatly on the unit that loses. The two units adjoin, and they freely share staff back and forth as the census demands. Jennifer and Jonathan brainstorm and come up with several options, such as rebidding the work based on two units that are adjacent (perhaps they could get a discount); renovating the units in phases, part one this year and part two the next; or perhaps if this was not possible, renovating one unit this year and purchasing new equipment for the other unit and then reversing the process. Jennifer and Jonathan make a joint appointment to speak with the Vice President of Nursing.

Case Study Questions

1. What type of conflict outcome were Jennifer and Jonathan attempting to elicit?
2. What types of conflict strategies were Jennifer and Jonathan using?
3. What type of framework for conflict strategy were Jennifer and Jonathan using to get their desired outcome?

LEARNING RESOURCES

Discussion Questions

1. Describe and discuss the three conflict resolution outcomes in terms of teambuilding and long-term positive relationships among individuals competing for resources.
2. Discuss the use of conflict resolution strategies, and identify the outcome possible when using each of the strategies.
3. How can nurses as a group work together to have significant impact on legislative issues affecting nursing practice?
4. Is collective bargaining useful in nursing? What is the purpose of collective bargaining and how can it be useful to nurses? How can it inhibit the nursing profession's growth?
5. What are sources of conflict in nursing and what can nurses do to resolve this conflict and promote growth?

Study Questions

True and False: Circle the correct answer.

T (F) 1. Conflict arises because job descriptions are clear, policies and procedures are written, and growth is fostered in an organization.

(T) F 2. Organizational conflict arises from the competition for scarce resources.

T (F) 3. In order to build effective interdisciplinary teams, conflict must be present, and managers must not interfere with conflict resolution.

T (F) 4. Role ambiguity is the expectation that nurses take on duties from other disciplines.

(T) F 5. People are most comfortable around people who are like them.

(T) F 6. A defensive framework for conflict resolution includes the winning of some resources and the loss of others.

(T) F 7. Using the conflict strategy of withdrawing provides the participant with the time to calm down or avoid confrontation.

T (F) 8. In a win-lose situation, both parties end up losing because nobody is one hundred percent satisfied.

(T) F 9. Collective bargaining is used by nurses to prevent management from making all of the decisions without input from the nurses about compensation and work load.

T (F) 10. Role stress occurs when the nurse's responsibilities expand faster than the formal job description.

SUPPLEMENTAL READINGS

Gardner, D.L. (1992). Conflict and retention of new graduate nurses. *Western Journal of Nursing Research, 14*(1), 76-85.

Pondy, L. (1967). Organizational conflict: Concepts and models. *Administrative Science Quarterly, 12,* 296-320.

Chapter 22

Persuasion and Negotiation

STUDY FOCUS

Conflict is inevitable. Nurses must learn effective strategies to resolve conflict and enhance collaborative efforts among interdisciplinary team members. Two powerful tools that may resolve conflicts are persuasion and negotiation. Individuals use persuasion to get what they want when they believe coercion is unethical. Bargaining and negotiation are also useful in resolving a conflict.

Persuasion is the ability to influence others to change their behavior based on argument or reasoning. An individual skillful at persuasion will leave the listener with some perception of choice. Persuaders have a variety of motives for their approach, with the most typical being self-preservation, money, romance, or recognition. Effective communication is essential when attempting to persuade others. In the course of persuasion, timing, strategy, and credibility are important in the attempt to lower listeners' defenses, as well as in complimenting, and supporting them. Commitment, imagination, and trust are three elements crucial to successful persuasion.

The five reasons for exerting influence are to obtain assistance, to get others to do their job, to obtain personal benefits, to initiate change, and to improve job performance. Assertiveness, ingratiation, rationality, sanctions, exchange, upward appeal, blocking, and coalitions are all influence tactics. In effective persuasion, two tactics are frequently used. They include the intensification of certain points and the downplaying other points. Important persuasive techniques are using repetition, creating miscommunication, and providing rational explanations, while avoiding threats and fear tactics.

Negotiation is the give-and-take exchange among individuals who want to resolve conflict in a way acceptable to all parties involved. Bargaining is closely related to negotiation and is the exchange of favors among individuals. Collective bargaining is a type of negotiation governed by specific laws and rules. Individuals engage in negotiation to prevent win-lose situations. In order to classify an interaction as a negotia-

tion, the following three criteria must be present: the issue must be negotiable; the negotiators must be willing to give and take; and the individuals must trust each other and the process. Four elements in the negotiation process are the goals, the values, mutual victory, and incomplete information.

There are ten steps in the negotiation process. The first step is preparing for the negotiation. The second step is communicating a general overview of what is to be accomplished in the negotiation. Third, the reasons why each party feels the negotiation is necessary should be reviewed. Fourth, the parties should redefine and clarify the issue(s). Fifth, the parties should agree on the agenda and select when in the course of meeting the issues will be addressed. In the sixth step, discussion should be encouraged and facilitated throughout the negotiation process. During discussions, the seventh step, an exploration of the compromise positions for both parties should be examined. Eighth, during the settlement stage, each party should agree in principle to the solution or possible solutions for the issue. Ninth, a thorough review and summarizing of the agreement should take place. Finally, a process should be established and implemented to monitor the parties' compliance and progress with the final agreement.

Formal negotiations have a specialized language that individuals use to convey the activities that occur throughout the process. Terms such as issues, deadlock or stalemate, impasse, concessions, power, flinch, deadline, nibble, and concessions are used. Issues refer to negotiable items or to those conflicts which need to be resolved. An impasse is a point in time when issues cannot be resolved. Impasses lead to deadlocks or stalemates in which individuals are unable to reach agreement. Concessions refer to favors given or positions changed in order to continue negotiations or to provide a satisfactory settlement to all parties. Power is the ability to influence others. A flinch is to express displeasure with the initial proposal in order to begin the negotiation process. A deadline is an end date on a schedule used to keep both parties on target and progressing in the negotiation process. The nibble is a small concession after the agreement has been settled. The concessions are those items that are of little or no value to you, but important to others and can be used strategically to influence the negotiation process.

Preparation for negotiations is essential and important for success. The ability to determine the parameters for negotiation helps control the issues and areas of discussion. Dressing professionally and being aware of both verbal and nonverbal messages are important in resolving issues and tipping off the opposing party. Good listening skills and a positive communication tone are essential for effective negotiation. Maintaining a position in which there is room for negotiation is also important in a successful negotiation.

Nurses have unionized for a variety of reasons. Some of the more recent issues sparking unionization efforts include layoffs, the reduction of hours, elimination of incentives, the cessation of pay increases, and the denial of benefits. The use of UAPs in place of RNs and the increasing number of employees a clinical nurse must supervise have sparked concerns about unsafe client care and inadequate staffing levels. To verbalize the concerns of nurses to management, nurses have occasionally turned to unionization as a method of strengthening their voice and demanding accountability for unilateral administrative decisions influencing client care. A recent blow to nursing's unionization activities came when the Supreme Court ruled in 1994 that nurses who supervise lower level personnel are considered supervisors and, therefore, are not afforded protection by the National Labor Relations Act.

LEARNING TOOLS

Role Play: #1

Using Persuasion to Influence Others

Character One = Jennifer is the vice president of nursing at a large teaching hospital in Topeka, Kansas. She has decided to organize a team to work on critical pathways and to then implement them in the hospital in an effort to provide cost-effective, high quality care to clients.

Character Two = Jason is the Chief Executive Officer (CEO) of the hospital. He is very concerned about rising costs and is tightening up on resources. He plans to hold the line and not distribute money for new projects that cannot guarantee a payoff.

Character Three = Joe is the vice president of building and maintenance. He is over budget on a new building project and needs additional moneys to finish the new building. He plans to speak to Jason to secure the needed funds.

Character Four = Mary Ann is the chief financial officer (CFO). She has crunched some figures and is prepared to speak to Jason about the bottom line. She has designed a forecasted projection of the next six months-revenue and expenses, and she is prepared to make recommendations about cost cutting to ensure organizational viability.

✦　✦　✦　✦

Jennifer has entered Jason's office prepared to share with him a new project (critical pathways) that would improve quality and decrease costs. She knows that there will be an initial outlay of money, but is sure that there will be a major payoff for the organization. As she turns the corner toward Jason's office, she sees Mary Ann and Joe talking. Jason opens his door and sees his executive team waiting to speak to him.

Role-play Questions:

1. What should Jennifer do? Should she take the lead and jump right in with her new idea? If so, what should she say? How should she introduce the topic?
2. What persuasive techniques should Jennifer use to elicit support for her project?
3. How could she persuade others to support her project and yet support them with their plans?

Role-play Worksheet

CHARACTERS	STUDENT ASSIGNED
Jennifer, The Vice President of Nursing	_____
Jason, The Chief Executive Officer	_____
Joe, The Vice President of Building and Maintenance	_____
Mary Ann, The Chief Financial Officer	_____

Role Play Assessment Questions

Which character have you been assigned?

What are your character's goals in this situation?

How can the other characters assist you in achieving your goals?

What might the other characters do to hinder you in achieving your goals?

What strategies and probes do you plan to use in this situation?

CASE STUDY

Jennifer is a nurse manager of an ambulatory care clinic in a large teaching hospital. The ambulatory care clinic is very successful and is a good revenue source for the hospital. Recently, the physicians and nurse practitioners in the ambulatory care clinic negotiated a contract with a large employer in the community to provide primary care for all of their employees. The contract was negotiated at a discounted rate, and so the physicians and nurse practitioners have held a team conference to look at expenses, workload, and equipment usage. They have asked Jennifer to figure out a way to use the RNs more effectively, and if necessary, to hire medical assistants. Jennifer knows that the nurses will be resistant. She also knows that the RNs could be utilized more effectively in client teaching activities, immunizations, and triage.

Case Study Questions

1. What should Jennifer do? Should she be autocratic and demand that the RNs comply? Should she use persuasion to get them to do what she wants? Should she negotiate with them?
2. If Jennifer chooses to use persuasion, should she listen to their concerns?
3. If Jennifer chooses to use negotiation and a settlement is agreed upon, who is responsible for evaluating and monitoring progress?

LEARNING RESOURCES

Discussion Questions

1. What are the current issues in healthcare organizations today that nurses might choose to unionize in order to have a strong collective voice?
2. Describe the process of negotiation that nurses could use to address pressing issues in client care with administrative personnel.
3. Are persuasion, negotiation and bargaining useful in both personal and professional interactions? If so, provide an example of each for both a personal and professional situation.
4. What is the difference between coercion and persuasion? Should both be used? If so, why? If not, why not?
5. Would you support unionization activities at your organization? If so, why? Are there other methods to resolve conflict? If so, what are they?

Study Questions

Matching: Write the letter of the correct response in front of each term.

_I_	1. negotiation
_J_	2. bargaining
_F_	3. persuasion
_E_	4. collective bargaining
_H_	5. flinch
_A_	6. nibble
_B_	7. concessions
_G_	8. deadline
_C_	9. impasses
_D_	10. issues

A. a small extra item that is obtained after the settlement

B. items of little value to one party

C. a point in time when issues cannot be resolved to mutual satisfaction

D. items to be resolved

E. activities governed by laws and rules

F. influencing another to modify behaviors

G. time frames for negotiations

H. to draw back at an initial proposal

I. give-and-take exchange aimed at resolving conflicts

J. the exchange of favors

SUPPLEMENTAL READINGS

Flarey, D.L., Yoder, S., & Barabas, M. (1992). Collaboration in labor relations: A model for success. *The Journal of Nursing Administration, 22*(9), 15-22.

Chapter 23

Staffing and Scheduling

STUDY FOCUS

Staffing and scheduling are important components in the effective provision of cost-effective, client-centered care and in the satisfaction, retention, and recruitment of nurses. Staffing is the development of a plan to hire qualified workers to fill designated positions in an organization. Scheduling is implementing the staffing pattern to assign workers to cover specific shifts and days on specific units. Staff mix is the skill level of workers that is required to provide care. Nursing resources include the number and types of workers designated to provide nursing services. The nursing workload is a compilation of nursing care needs of clients. Acuity is the intensity or severity of client illness. Nursing intensity is the amount and complexity of care required by clients. A nurse extender is a worker who completes designated tasks in order to assist the nurses to care for a larger number of clients or to offer clients a broader selection of services.

Staffing decisions are complex and require planning and careful consideration for maximum effectiveness. Four essential elements of staffing decisions include a statement of philosophy, general objectives for the department and specific objectives for the unit, job descriptions for all skill levels, and a statement of the frequency of nursing care along with a designation of who will provide the services. Typically, staffing decisions are based on a measure of volume and/or time. Volume measures include census, visits, births, operations, and client contacts. One method of volume calculation is hours per patient day (HPPD). HPPD is a calculation of nursing hours needed per unit of service.

Two methods used to guide nurse staffing are fixed and variable staffing. Fixed staffing is a fixed maximum workload requirement. This type of staffing method is based on the assumption that one will have maximum workload conditions. Variable staffing is based on a supplementary approach and involves staffing below maximum workload conditions. A proposed third type of staffing method is a semiflexible system whereby 15% of the staff are fixed. In semiflexible staffing, the fixed staff are supplemented based on volume and acuity.

There are eleven steps in designing a staffing pattern. First, select criteria to determine the intensity levels of clients or units of service. Second, determine the time required to complete the work. The third step is to collect data to determine the validity of a set classification system. Fourth, collect sufficient data (type and quantity) to evaluate your proposed staffing method. Fifth, determine the average number of minutes per activity or task. The sixth step is to establish a performance time for new functions. Seventh, decide on the staff mix necessary to complete the work. Eighth, determine the amount of time per client type necessary (severity of illness) for each skill level. Ninth, establish a projected unit of service projection for the year. The tenth step is to calculate the total number of nursing hours and the number of individuals by skill mix that will be needed per year. Finally, designate the number of individuals per shift each day and their skill mix. Include a calculation for time off and administrative activities.

Many types of client classification systems are in use today. The three broad types of client classification systems include prototype, factor, and computerized real-time factor. A prototype client classification system is designed to categorize clients by broad categories and characteristics. The factor client classification system uses critical indicators to determine individual care needs. In the factor systems, allowances are made for the indirect care activities required. The computerized real-time factor systems are based on actual care requirements for individual clients.

Differentiated nursing practice is a philosophy of nursing roles, functions, and work based on education, experience, and competence. Four tiers of differentiated practice are general healthcare aides, nurse professionals who handle emerging patterns, nurse professionals who handle complex changes, and nurse professionals who develop a knowledge base. The educational preparation of nurses is diverse ranging from a diploma to a baccalaureate degree. The use of nurse extenders (NEs) has created much controversy in the nursing profession. As hospitals redesign and restructure client-centered delivery care systems, the number and role of nurse extenders has expanded. There are concerns that nurse extenders are not adequately trained to perform multiple tasks and therefore compromise quality care.

LEARNING TOOLS

Activity: Staffing and Scheduling

Purpose: To become familiar with the staffing and scheduling process.

Introduction: Staffing a unit in a hospital or ambulatory care clinic is a challenging process. A manager must assess employees' requests for time off which include vacation, scheduled days off, and personal time. They must also handle the call-ins for sick time. To effectively staff a unit, the manager must establish a skill-mix level and project a unit service figure. The activity below provides you an opportunity to staff a unit and see the complexities of scheduling and staffing.

Staffing and Scheduling Scenario:
B6–Oncology unit (25 beds)
Average daily census 17
Skill mix: 75% RNs
25% NEs

The nurse manager has determined that ten staff are required for a 24-hour period. The nurse manager must cover 24 hours per week for 7 days a week. The breakdown for % of nurses needed is: days–45%, evening–36%, and nights–19%

Employees: RNs: Susie is full-time (7-3); Jen is full-time (7-3); Jon is full-time (7-3); Sylvia is full-time (7-3); Ben is full-time (7-3 and 3-11); Jake is full-time (3-11); Kim is full-time (3-11); Cindy is 24 hours per week (3-11); Jack is a prn and works on an as-needed basis (3-11 and 11-7); Tom is full-time (11-7); and Jan is full-time (11-7).

NEs: Jill is full-time (7-3); Joan is 24 hours per week (7-3); Jeremy is prn (3-11); Jerry is part-time 24 hours per week (3-11); Janet is prn (3-11); and Jessie is 32 hours per week (11-7). It is important to hire some prn or pool nurses who are flexible to assist in meeting vacation coverage.

RN requests: Susie cannot work Mondays because of school. Jen is getting married and needs September 1-17 off for her honeymoon. Jon is going away for a fishing trip and needs the first weekend of September off. Jack does not want to work Tuesdays and Thursdays because of babysitting difficulties and does not want every weekend.

NE requests: Jessie will be on vacation September 1-10. Janet will not be able to work Fridays because of a continuing education course.

Directions: Create a schedule with the following requests using the census of 17, and calculate the number of staff needed per shift. First determine how many employees are on each shift — day, evening, and night shifts. Then calculate the number of RNs and NEs needed per day, evening, and night shifts. Next, put all the requests on your calendar. Finally, create a schedule, using the empty schedule grid on the following page (remember, employees do not like working every weekend).

Questions to Consider

1. How many employees will be scheduled for each shift?
2. What type of employees will be scheduled for each shift? How many of each skill level?
3. Are there any vacation or personal requests?
4. Who works full time and who works part time? What are the part time employees' hours?

Schedule for September 1995

September 7–3 shift

	F	S	S	M	T	W	Th	F	S	S	M	T	W	Th	F	S	S	M	T	W	Th	F	S	S	M	T	W	Th	F	S
	1	2	3	4	5	6	7	8	9	10	11	12	13	14	15	16	17	18	19	20	21									
RNs Susie (FT)																														
Jen (FT)																														
Jon (FT)																														
Sylvia (FT)																														
Ben (FT)																														
NEs Jill (FT)																														
Joan (PT)																														
Jeremy (PRN)																														

September 3–11 shift

| **RNs** Jake (FT) |
| Kim (FT) |
| Cindy (PT) |
| **NEs** Jerry (PT) |
| Janet (PRN) |

September 11–7 shift

| Tom (FT) |
| Jan (FT) |
| **RNs** Jack (PRN) |
| **NEs** Jessie (PT) |

Jessie
Sep 1 – 10 – vacation

40 ✓
40 ✓
no T or Th ✓
32 ✓
4 shifts/wk

Summary: Working with staffing and scheduling is complex. When people call in due to illness or personal crisis, finding fill ins can be harrowing. Meeting individual requests in a tight schedule can be problematic. Many units have resorted to self-scheduling to give staff more flexibility to plan their work and personal lives and to encourage them to covere each other's shifts.

One Possible Solution: There should be 5 staff on 7-3, 3 on 3-11, and 2 on 11-7. Next, calculate how many RNs and NEs should be scheduled per shift. On 7-3, there should be 4 RNs/1 NE; on 3-11 there should be 2 RNs/1 NE; and on 11-7 there should be 1 RN/1 NE. Nurse managers have the flexibility to shift the total number of RNs and NEs within the 24-hours shift, and at times, they may alter the skill mix throughout the year to cover vacations and requests. The key is to keep salaries averaging out over the year (remember, a nurse manager budgets salaries based on the number of RNs and NEs working per shift). Many times, weekends are typically staffed with fewer nurses in order to allow staff members every other weekend off. Following is a sample of a completed schedule based on the situation described.

Schedule for September 1995

September 7–3 shift

	F 1	S 2	S 3	M 4	T 5	W 6	Th 7	F 8	S 9	S 10	M 11	T 12	W 13	Th 14	F 15	S 16	S 17	M 18	T 19	W 20	Th 21	F 22	S 23	S 24	M 25	T 26	W 27	Th 28	F 29	S 30
RNs Susie (FT)	7–3	7–3	7–3	X	X	7–3	7–3	X	7–3	7–3	X	7–3	7–3	7–3	7–3	X	X	X	7–3	7–3	7–3	X	7–3	7–3	X	7–3	7–3	7–3	7–3	X
Jen (FT)	VAC	X	X	VAC	VAC	VAC	VAC	VAC	X	X	VAC	VAC	VAC	VAC	VAC	X	X	7–3	7–3	7–3	X	7–3	7–3	7–3	7–3	X	X	7–3	7–3	7–3
Jon (FT)	7–3	X	X	7–3	7–3	VAC	VAC	VAC	7–3	7–3	VAC	VAC	VAC	VAC	VAC	7–3	7–3	7–3	7–3	7–3	X	7–3	7–3	7–3	X	7–3	7–3	7–3	7–3	7–3
Sylvia (FT)	7–3	7–3	7–3	X	7–3	7–3	X	7–3	X	7–3	7–3	7–3	7–3	X	7–3	7–3	7–3	7–3	7–3	X	7–3	7–3	X	X	7–3	7–3	X	X	7–3	7–3
Ben (FT)	X	3–11	7–3	7–3	7–3	X	7–3	7–3	7–3	7–3	3–11	X	7–3	7–3	7–3	7–3	7–3	X	X	7–3	7–3	X	7–3	7–3	7–3	7–3	X	7–3	7–3	3–11
NEs Jill (FT)	7–3	7–3	7–3	7–3	X	X	7–3	7–3	7–3	X	7–3	7–3	X	7–3	7–3	X	7–3	X	7–3	7–3	7–3	7–3	X	7–3	7–3	7–3	7–3	7–3	X	7–3
Joan (PT)	7–3	7–3	X	7–3	X	X	7–3	7–3	X	7–3	7–3	7–3	7–3	7–3	X	7–3	7–3	7–3	X	X	7–3	X	X	X	7–3	X	7–3	X	X	7–3
Jeremy (PRN)	X	X	X	7–3	7–3	7–3	X	7–3	7–3	7–3	7–3	X	X	7–3	X	7–3	X	7–3	X	X	X	7–3	X	X	X	X	7–3	X	X	X

September 3–11 shift

	F 1	S 2	S 3	M 4	T 5	W 6	Th 7	F 8	S 9	S 10	M 11	T 12	W 13	Th 14	F 15	S 16	S 17	M 18	T 19	W 20	Th 21	F 22	S 23	S 24	M 25	T 26	W 27	Th 28	F 29	S 30
RNs Jake (FT)	3–11	X	X	3–11	3–11	3–11	X	3–11	3–11	3–11	X	3–11	3–11	3–11	3–11	X	X	3–11	3–11	3–11	X	3–11	3–11	3–11	X	3–11	3–11	3–11	3–11	X
Kim (FT)	3–11	3–11	3–11	X	3–11	3–11	3–11	3–11	X	X	3–11	3–11	X	3–11	3–11	3–11	3–11	3–11	3–11	3–11	3–11	3–11	X	3–11	3–11	3–11	3–11	3–11	3–11	3–11
Cindy (PT)	X	X	X	3–11	3–11	X	3–11	3–11	3–11	3–11	X	3–11	3–11	3–11	3–11	3–11	X	3–11	3–11	X	3–11	X	3–11	3–11	3–11	X	X	3–11	3–11	X
NEs Jerry (PT)	3–11	X	X	3–11	X	3–11	X	X	3–11	3–11	X	X	3–11	X	X	X	3–11	3–11	X	X	3–11	X	3–11	3–11	3–11	3–11	3–11	X	X	X
Janet (PRN)	X	3–11	3–11	X	7–3	7–3	3–11	X	X	X	3–11	X	X	X	X	3–11	3–11	X	X	X	X	X	X	3–11	3–11	X	X	X	X	3–11

September 11–7 shift

	F 1	S 2	S 3	M 4	T 5	W 6	Th 7	F 8	S 9	S 10	M 11	T 12	W 13	Th 14	F 15	S 16	S 17	M 18	T 19	W 20	Th 21	F 22	S 23	S 24	M 25	T 26	W 27	Th 28	F 29	S 30
Tom (FT)	11–7	11–7	X	11–7	11–7	11–7	11–7	X	11–7	11–7	11–7	X	11–7	11–7	11–7	X	X	11–7	11–7	11–7	11–7	X	11–7	11–7	11–7	X	11–7	11–7	11–7	X
Jan (FT)	11–7	11–7	11–7	X	11–7	11–7	11–7	11–7	X	X	11–7	11–7	X	11–7	11–7	11–7	11–7	11–7	11–7	11–7	11–7	11–7	X	X	11–7	X	X	11–7	11–7	11–7
RNs Jack (PRN)	X	X	11–7	11–7	X	X	11–7	11–7	11–7	11–7	X	X	11–7	X	X	X	11–7	X	X	X	X	3–11	X	X	X	11–7	X	X	X	11–7
NEs Jessie (PT)	VAC	X	X	VAC	VAC	VAC	VAC	VAC	X	X	11–7	11–7	11–7	11–7	X	X	11–7	11–7	X	X	X	11–7	11–7	11–7	X	11–7	11–7	X	X	X

CASE STUDY

Dorothy, a graduate prepared nurse manager of a 79-bed medical unit, decides to operationalize differentiated nursing practice in order to maximize the use of each nurses skills and knowledge base. The medical unit is staffed by nurse's aides, licensed practical nurses, diploma, associate degree, baccalaureate, and graduate prepared nurses. Dorothy conducts a literature review to obtain pertinent information and to review successful models of differentiated nursing practice. Then Dorothy seeks volunteers to form a task force to modify job descriptions and examine compensation levels for differentiated practice.

Case Study Questions

1. Is it possible to establish a staffing plan based on a differentiated practice model?
2. What might be the basis for differentiating practice?
3. Is it appropriate to compensate nurses based on differentiated practice? If so why? If not why not?

LEARNING RESOURCES

Discussion Questions

1. What factors make staffing and scheduling complex?
2. Should clinical nurses have a say in scheduling? If so, why? If not, why not? Should there be scheduling parameters established by the administration? Or should clinical nurses establish their own scheduling guidelines?
3. How do you calculate HHPD? Is this a useful calculation?
4. What must be considered when developing a client classification system?
5. What are the three broad types of client classification and what are the differences and similarities among them?

Study Questions

True and False: Circle the correct answer.

T   F   1. Staffing is the implementation of a staffing pattern indicating the number and type of workers to be scheduled per shift.

T   F   2. Variable staffing is based upon a set maximum workload requirement.

T   F   3. Client classification is the grouping of clients according to nursing care requirements.

T   F   4. Differentiated nursing practice uses criteria such as education, experience, and competence.

T   F   5. Restructuring has enhanced nursing practice and increased the need for RNs in hospitals.

T   F   6. Nurse extenders assist nurses to perform client care tasks including vital signs and assessments.

T   F   7. Acuity is the severity of a client illness.

T   F   8. Components in determining the severity of illness include client dependency, complexity, the time to complete tasks, and the skill level of the worker needed.

T   F   9. Staffing decisions are based solely on an individual's philosophy.

T   F   10. Nursing workload is the number of client days and the hours of nursing care required per client day.

SUPPLEMENTAL READINGS

Warren, I. & Rozell , B. (1995). Supplemental staffing: Nurse manager views of costs, benefits, and quality of care. *The Journal of Nursing Administration, 25*(6), 51-57.

Jung, F., Pearcey, L., & Phillips, J. (1994). Evaluation of a program to improve nursing assistant use. *The Journal of Nursing Administration, 24*(3), 42-47.

Chapter 24

Computer Applications in Nursing Administration

STUDY FOCUS

Computer applications in nursing administration are crucial to effect decision making for effective quality client care. Nursing must establish a standardized nursing data base in order to make meaningful comparisons across sites. Computer applications have provided an efficient and effective method of acquiring financial data to evaluate outcomes of care.

Computers are the tools for managing data. Informatics is a combination of computer and information science. Nursing informatics is the management of nursing data, information, and knowledge as it is applied to nursing care delivery. Effectiveness research is the use of large data sets applying epidemiological methods to evaluate relationships. Management information systems (MIS) are integrated to collect, store, retrieve, and process data. Ten criteria for an effective MIS are the following: informative, relevant, sensitive, unbiased, comprehensive, timely, action-oriented, uniform, performance-targeted, and cost-effective.

The standardization of a nursing data set is essential to capture the contributions that nurses make to client care. Reimbursement decisions are made based on hard data that is easily retrievable and that show positive outcomes. Four domains of nursing's data needs include the client data, provider data, administrative data, and research data. Nurses must clearly define their data elements, identify linkages between and among data sets, and design a clear coding system to ensure usable data sets. The determination of data elements and engineering technology are important aspects of nursing informatics.

Large data bases are now being developed to collect information on healthcare workers and client care. Examples include the Institute of Medicine's Computer-based Patient Record of an account of client care and the American Nurses' Association's Nursing Information System (NIS), which keeps records of nurses' licensure and credentials. There are many advantages to large data sets, but there are also limitations. Problems can include flawed data, inadequate methodologies, and the misuse of sensitive healthcare information on practitioner practice patterns.

The end result of computerized applications to nursing administration for nurse leaders is the designing of an integrated management information system that uses standardized nursing language and data elements for comparative purposes. To advocate the inclusion of essential nursing data elements in national data bases is crucial for nursing practice and reimbursement. The Uniform Hospital Discharge Data Set does not include nursing data elements because nursing lacks a standardized data set that is clearly defined, valid, and reliable. Nurses are challenged to identify and validate a standardized nursing data set to ensure inclusion in national data sets. Such efforts are currently underway for nursing administration. The Nursing Management Minimum Data Set (NMMDS) is a data base that includes service-related management data elements. Data elements include cost, quality, and outcome data. The limitations of the NMMDS are that nursing practice and personnel data about individual nurses is omitted, and it lacks uniform collection practices across sites.

LEARNING TOOLS

Activity: Domains of Nursing Data

Purpose: To identify essential elements in the four domains of nursing data.

Directions: Using the following spaces for each of the four domains of nursing data listed, identify elements in each domain that would be important to collect and analyze in a NIS. Review Table 24.1 in the Huber text on p. 470 for outcomes and variables in the three domains of nursing data needs, and review Table

24.2 on p. 476 of the Huber text for proposed NMMDS elements. These two tables will give you ideas about essential data elements for each of the four domains.

1. Client: clinical data and outcomes
   Source: client record

   _____

   _____

   _____

   _____

2. Provider: professional data, caregiver outcomes, and decision-maker variables
   Source: personnel records, data banks, and client records

   _____

   _____

   _____

   _____

3. Administrative: systems outcomes, contextual variables, administrative data
   Source: management data and fiscal data sources

   _____

   _____

   _____

   _____

4. Research: knowledge base information
   Source: existing and new data and regional databases

   _____

   _____

   _____

   _____

Each of the four nursing domains are important to include in NIS and MIS. Identifying essential variables and outcome by nursing unit and by institution is critical in obtaining quantifiable comparable data. This data can be used to compare units within an institution as well as across institutions. The collection and analysis of basic nursing data sets are important for nursing to demonstrate nurses' unique contribution to client care.

CASE STUDY

Jackie is a nursing director of critical care and has been asked to make recommendations for purchasing a nursing information system (NIS) for a large teaching hospital. Jackie is very knowledgeable about clinical issues, but has not had much experience with computers or information systems. Jackie reads about NIS and MIS and wonders if purchasing an MIS would not be a better choice for the organization. She struggles to determine which data elements are essential when purchasing an NIS.

Case Study Questions

1. Would an MIS meet the needs of a nurse administrator?
2. Is there an advantage to a nurse administrator in purchasing an NIS over an MIS?
3. What four domains of nursing data should Jackie remember to include as criteria for selection of an NIS?

LEARNING RESOURCES

Discussion Questions

1. What is the difference between informatics and nursing informatics?
2. What is effectiveness research and how can it be useful in nursing practice?
3. How can standardized nursing data sets help nurses gain reimbursement status for nursing services?
4. Should the NMMDS be refined or should a new data set be designed? Why?
5. Identify benefits of an NIS for clinical nurses. Identify any barriers for clinical nurses in using an NIS.

Study Questions

Matching: Write the letter of the correct response in front of each term.

_____ 1. nursing informatics

_____ 2. informatics

_____ 3. computer

_____ 4. effectiveness research

_____ 5. management information system

_____ 6. Computer-based patient record

_____ 7. NMMDS

_____ 8. quality improvement tools

A. tool for managing data

B. analysis of large data bases using epidemiological methods

C. combination of computer and information science

D. integrated system to collect and manipulate data for the purposes of directing and controlling resources

E. management of data to support the practice and delivery of nursing care

F. tracks longitudinal accounts of client care

G. identifies common causes of variation and visual display of data

H. elements crucial to evaluation of nursing interventions on client outcomes

SUPPLEMENTAL READINGS

Ferrand, D. & Lay, C. (1994). Diagnosing strategic performance of the hospital information systems planning cycle. *Health Care Management Review, 19*(3), 21-33.

Lieberg, S. (1995). Computerized nursing management systems: 4M's for maintenance. *Nursing Management, 26*(3), 29-30.

Nadzam, D. & Cole, K. (1994). The joint commission's indicator measurement system: Implications for information systems. *Healthcare Information Management, 8*(2), 13-21.

Chapter 25

Quality Improvement and Risk Management

STUDY FOCUS

Quality improvement is an essential component of healthcare and is linked with evaluation and accountability. There is tremendous pressure on healthcare organizations to deliver high quality care at lower costs in order to compete successfully in a competitive environment. Quality is the provision of excellent care that is effective, efficient, and appropriate. Quality of care refers to the delivery of healthcare services and the belief that using up-to-date professional knowledge will likely result in positive outcomes. Assurance is the completion of services in an excellent manner. Quality assurance is the provision of services according to professional standards in a manner acceptable to the client. Quality improvement programs are implemented organizationwide to ensure accountability to clients and payers. Total quality process or total quality management is a method of including all employees in the improvement of services to ensure client satisfaction. Continuous quality improvement is a multidisciplinary process to improve systems by analyzing performance, collecting data, and changing archaic or inefficient systems.

Cost, equity, access, and quality considerations underlie healthcare policies and decisions. Quality assessment (measurement) activities began in the l880s with Florence Nightingale collecting data and developing standards. Quality assessment has evolved from close scrutiny and the monitoring of quality indicators (quality assurance) to the systemwide implementation of multdisciplinary teams in a continuous effort to improve systems (total quality improvement). Trends in quality improvement include the development of interdisciplinary quality assurance teams, client satisfaction, quality circles and councils, and the automation of quality indicators.

W. Edward Deming was influential in alerting Americans to the necessity of commitment to quality and listening to the customer's concerns. He used a unit-based approach focused on using higher quality to entice loyal customers. Key principles necessary for continuous quality improvement include organizational commitment, on understanding of individual client needs, a continuously improving process, commitment to high quality services, the use of data, commitment by top management, benchmarking, and the formation of long-term relationships with a few suppliers.

Regulatory agencies impact organizational standards and quality by establishing minimal levels for compliance. The Joint Commission on Accreditation of Healthcare Organizations (JCAHO) accredits healthcare organizations in ambulatory care, long-term care, psychiatric care, home care, and hospitals. Without accreditation, Medicare and Medicaid reimbursement will not be paid to a healthcare agency. The JCAHO ten-step process for quality assurance includes assigning responsibility, delineating the scope of practice, identifying important aspects of care, designating specific indicators of care, establishing thresholds for evaluation, collecting data, evaluating care, acting to solve problems, assessing actions and documenting improvement, and communicating quality.

Standards are established by professional organizations and regulatory agencies and can be written in terms of structure, process, or outcomes. Structural standards focus on the internal organization and its personnel. Process standards measure activities, and outcome standards measure whether the services made a difference. A standard of care is outcome-oriented and identifies what the client can expect. A standard of practice is process-oriented and identifies what the provider must do to achieve the standard of care.

Standards are measured by audits, which may be concurrent or retrospective. Concurrent audits are ongoing while the client is receiving services; whereas, retrospective audits occur after the services are provided. Documentation is the core source of audits. Commonly used tools to illustrate data in a logical manner include flow charts, fishbone diagrams, and pareto charts. Research and quality assessment are both evaluation techniques. Research is highly controlled and experimental. Quality assessment is day-to-day evaluation. Research is intended to be generalizable, but quality assurance is to determine effectiveness, efficiency, and appropriateness of care. Quality assurance evaluation tends to identify researchable problems, while research can strengthen a quality improvement program.

Professions monitor their own practice to set standards and ensure public accountability. Many professions require ongoing continuing education as a mechanism to ensure that their members stay current. Risk management programs are organizational methods of identifying risks, controlling occurrences, preventing damage, and controlling legal liability. The goal of risk management departments is to minimize financial loss due to malpractice claims. Risk management activities are focused on high-risk behaviors or areas in an attempt to prevent accidents. Organizations typically use incident reports to determine high-risk activities, track them, and implement control programs to prevent further occurrences.

LEARNING TOOLS

Activity: Organizational Quality Improvement Assessment

Purpose: To assess the level of continuous quality improvement in the organization in which you work.

Directions: Read each statement below, and then circle the number that best describes your assessment.

Key: 1–not at all, 2–to a small extent, 3–to a moderate extent, 4–to a great extent, and 5–to a very great extent

1. Employees clearly understand who the customer is.   1 2 3 4 5
2. All employees clearly understand the customer's needs.   1 2 3 4 5
3. There is regular contact with the customer.   1 2 3 4 5
4. There is ongoing quality assessment about the customer's needs and what is actually provided.   1 2 3 4 5
5. Employees work in interdisciplinary team.   1 2 3 4 5
6. Employees independently identify problems and seek to improve them.   1 2 3 4 5
7. Employees handle customer complaints autonomously.   1 2 3 4 5
8. Employees are valued and treated with respect.   1 2 3 4 5
9. Employees are allowed to do what it takes to do a high-quality job.   1 2 3 4 5
10. Employees are encouraged to handle work problems.   1 2 3 4 5
11. Employees do not need managerial approval to handle problems.   1 2 3 4 5
12. Experimentation and risk taking is valued and encouraged.   1 2 3 4 5
13. Change is viewed positively by employees.   1 2 3 4 5
14. Employees are encouraged to meet and discuss work.   1 2 3 4 5
15. Employees feel free to discuss matters openly and have no fear about disagreeing or offering alternative solutions.   1 2 3 4 5
16. Failures are viewed as learning opportunities and not punished.   1 2 3 4 5
17. Managers facilitate employees' work and encourage input into work activities and consumer needs.   1 2 3 4 5
18. Communication is open, and employees are kept informed of changes.   1 2 3 4 5
19. Group members work cohesively and share recognition for team accomplishments.   1 2 3 4 5
20. Individuals in top management positions are visible and encourage employee input into organizational matters.   1 2 3 4 5
21. Employees enjoy and have fun at work.   1 2 3 4 5
22. Innovation is encouraged, facilitated, and supported.   1 2 3 4 5

Scoring: Add up the total score for all 22 items. The higher the score the more apt your organization is to have a quality improvement program or strong elements of a program in place. Organizations that have continuous quality improvement programs tend to value employees, satisfy customers, and continually improve the process and services provided. Innovations are prized and risk taking is encouraged.

CASE STUDY

Pat is a Master's prepared nurse who has been asked by the Chief Executive Officer (CEO) of a medium-sized community hospital in Waterloo, Tennessee, to develop an organizationwide program to monitor major occurrences. Pat knows that there is an incident report system currently in place at the hospital, but the only people who see the reports are the managers. Pat decides to centralize the incident report system, identify and track major occurrences, and develop programs to minimize incidents. Pat decides to create a task force composed of employees and managers to relate her concerns and to elicit feedback. The CEO has informed Pat that one of her responsibilities was to decrease the amount and number of malpractice claims.

Case Study Questions

1. What type of program is Pat designing?
2. Is the program Pat is designing a component of quality improvement?
3. Should incident reports be used in a punitive manner?

LEARNING RESOURCES

Discussion Questions

1. Describe what continuous quality improvement (CQI) is, and identify key elements of a CQI program.
2. What are the similarities and differences in quality assessment and research?
3. What is the ten-step process of quality assurance for organizations as outlined by the Joint Commission on Accreditation of Healthcare Organizations (JCAHO)?
4. Why do healthcare organizations seek accreditation from JCAHO?
5. What is the difference between a standard of care and a standard of practice?

Study Questions

True or False: Circle the correct answer.

T F 1. A standard of care is outcome-oriented and focuses on the nurse as a provider.

T F 2. The three areas in which quality can be measured are structure, process, and cost.

T F 3. A feature of a profession is that it monitors its own practice.

T F 4. Risk management programs are designed to assure a high level of quality.

T F 5. Once an incident report is filled out, it absolves the person from responsibility for the occurrence.

T F 6. Standards can only be set by professional organizations.

T F 7. Retrospective audits are popular because an organization can monitor the client's progress while he is receiving services.

T F 8. Today, emphasis is on outcomes rather than process.

T F 9. Continuous quality improvement aims to develop long-term relationships with a few suppliers and is responsive to customer needs.

T F 10. Quality assurance is a highly controlled experimental research of client services.

SUPPLEMENTAL READINGS

Bedwell, R.T., Jr. (1993). How to adopt total quality managment: Laying a sound foundation. *Nonprofit World, 11*(4), 28-34.

Bedwell, R.T., Jr. (1993). Total quality managment: Making the decision. *Nonprofit World, 11*(3), 29-31.

Chapter **26**

Management of Change

STUDY FOCUS

Change is described as a process that is inevitable in our personal and professional lives. Change is the process of making something different. Change ranges on a continuum from haphazard to planned. Planned change is intentional intervention. A change agent is an individual that may be used to assist with planning and implementing change. The three strategies for organizational change are the rational-empirical, the normative-reeducative, and the power-coercive. The four areas in which organizational change may occur in nursing today include the organizational structures, the nursing labor force, reimbursement, and information systems. Change has been described by nursing leaders as a ruthless force capable of destroying those who refuse to adapt (O'Malley, 1995).

Part of planning change is examining the situational elements of organizational structure, people, and resources before implementing a change strategy. Four influences on change are individuals, face-to-face groups, organizations, and communities. Many theories can be used to facilitate the change process. The most widely used theory is Lewin's change theory. Lewin provides a framework from which a force field analysis is conducted. The three elements of his theory are unfreezing, moving, and refreezing. Unfreezing, a process in which individuals become ready to change, occurs first. During the unfreezing process, individuals become aware of unmet expectations and feel discomfort over action or inaction causing them to remove obstacles to change. The second stage is moving, which is when cognitive redefinition occurs. During the moving phase, a pretrial or testing occurs. The final stage, refreezing, is when the change occurs and is integrated and stabilized. During refreezing, leaders provide positive feedback, encouragement, and motivation to reinforce the new change.

There are many other change theories including Rogers's, who proposed that both the background of the individuals and the environment are antecedents to change. Rogers identified five phases of the change process — awareness, interest, evaluation, trial, and adoption. He believes that individuals choose one of two outcomes. They either accept and adopt the change, or they reject it. Another theory is Lippitt's who expanded Lewin's work by describing seven phases of change — diagnosing the problem, assessing motivation and the capacity to change, assessing motivation and resources, selecting change objectives, choosing roles for change agents, maintaining change, and terminating the helping relationship with the change agent. A fourth theory is Havelock's, who identified a planned change process with six elements — building relationships, diagnosing problems, acquiring resources, choosing solutions, gaining acceptance, and finally stabilizing and self-renewal.

Individuals respond differently to change. Some individuals are exhilarated while others are depressed, confused, and angry. Being aware of the emotional responses to a change can assist leaders to manage and facilitate change in a positive manner. Perlman and Takas (1990) identified the ten stages of the emotional voyage during change. The ten stages ar equilibrium, denial, anger, bargaining, chaos, depression, resignation, openness, readiness, and reemergence. Resistance is another important characteristic of individuals experiencing the change process. Resistance occurs for many different reasons. Some individuals are afraid of disorder and the interruption of their daily routine, while others are fearful of losing their job, power, or resources. Resistance can be useful if structured positively. Encouraging individuals to discuss change openly and to identify opportunities and barriers can create a smooth transition.

Leadership is necessary during change. Effective leaders have good diagnostic skills and the ability to adapt the leadership style to the situation and change some or all of the situational variables during the change process. Ineffective change elements include defensiveness, giving advice, and premature persuasion. Allowing participants in the change process the opportunity to verbalize their concerns is important. One can increase the effectiveness of change by explaining the rationale for change, allowing emotions to be expressed, giving participants information, and helping individuals with the change.

Innovations are the creation of something new. Innovation often entails a systematic, purposeful, and organized search for solutions to existing problems. Careful analysis and research occur prior to innovation. Sources of innovation include the following: examining the unexpected, incongruity, process needs, changes in industry or market structure, demographics, new knowledge, and change in perceptions or moods (Drucker 1992). McCloskey, et. al. (1994) identified five types of nursing innovations — introducing new technology, creating personnel development strategies, changing the organization of work, changing rewards/incentives, and implementing quality improvement mechanisms.

LEARNING TOOLS

Activity

Purpose: To examine and use a change theory evaluation instrument to assess the utility of a specific change theory for your desired change.

Introduction: Change is inevitable, occurring continuously in our daily lives. By taking charge of change and planning change activities, you can maintain control over a turbulent environment. Many change theories are in the literature. By evaluating the theory you wish to use with a specific planned change, you will have a clear sense of the utility of the change theory for your desired change. The following tool will assist you with evaluating change theories.

Identify a pet project that you would like to institute at work. Select a planned change theory that you would like to use to assess the readiness for the change, guide the process of change, and assist you at the evaluation of the change. Huber text pp. 513-516 describes several change theories. Use the Tiffany/Lutjens Planned Change Theory Evaluation Instrument to assess the utility of the change theory for your pet project.

The Tiffany/Lutjens Planned Change Theory Evaluation Instrument

The scoring for this tool is 0 for "I fully disagree" to 4 for "I fully agree".

0   I fully disagree
1
2
3
4   I fully agree

Directions: Choose a change theory. Write a number from 0 to 4 on the line in front of the statement that reflects your beliefs about the utility of this theory to your specific change.

I. Significance

_____   1. The planned change theory addresses targets for change.

_____   2. This theory has an assessment process that could help a change agent identify a problem in a social system.

_____   3. The theory has a clear process for evaluating the total change event.

_____   4. The theory accounts for emerging problems and/or goals throughout the change process.

_____   5. The theory prompts nursing change agents to ask if the proposed change is important for nursing.

_____   6. The theory encourages the ethical use of power.

_____   7. The theory encourages close cooperation between change agents and target populations.

_____   8. The theory encourages change agents to help people in the target population make informed decisions.

_____   9. The theory stresses social justice.

_____   10. The theory looks at the world as a whole.

_____   11. The theory views the world as changing rather than nonchanging.

_____   12. The theory prompts change agents to consider whether the strategies they plan will agree with expectations of the social unit targeted for change.

II. Clarity and Consistency

_____   13. This theory has a clear process for planning change.

_____   14. This theory has a clear process for implementing change (causing change to occur).

_____   15. This theory clearly defines planned change.

_____   16. The definition of planned change fits with the remainder of the content of the theory.

_____   17. Key ideas are clearly defined.

_____   18. Relational statements are clearly stated.

_____   19. Key ideas and relational statements avoid unnecessary repetition.

_____   20. Key ideas are consistently used as defined throughout the theory

____ 21. The theory clearly states what it accepts as truth (assumptions).

____ 22. Key ideas are related to one another.

____ 23. Any diagrams offered increase the reader's understanding of planned change and its processes.

____ 24. The planned change theory contributes to an understanding of planned change beyond what could be obtained from everyday experience or formal study of other planned change theories.

III. Generality

____ 25. The planned change theory could help agents plan change.

____ 26. The theory focuses only on the processes of planned change, not on unplanned change.

____ 27. The purpose of the theory allows a change agent to carry out plans for change in any one of a number of clinical settings rather than in one specific setting or area.

____ 28. This theory could apply to individuals.

____ 29. This theory could apply to groups.

____ 30. This theory could apply to communities.

____ 31. This theory could apply to society.

____ 32. This theory could apply to different cultures both within and outside the United States.

____ 33. Nurses could use this theory as a foundation for research.

____ 34. The theory could be tested through research.

____ 35. Hypotheses that can be tested could be developed from the theory.

____ 36. Key ideas and processes of the theory can be observed in the real world.

IV. Practicality

____ 37. The theory prompts change agents to consider time frames.

____ 38. The theory prompts change agents to consider the people (including experts) available to make the change.

____ 39. The theory prompts change agents to consider space, equipment, and supplies.

____ 40. The theory prompts change agents to consider financial resources.

____ 41. The theory prompts change agents to consider organizational support.

____ 42. The theory promotes change agents to consider whether they can obtain needed political resources for implementing change.

____ 43. The theory prompts change agents to consider whether they can obtain needed legal resources for implementing change.

V. Applicability

____ 44. Nurse change agents could use this theory to create change in clinical settings.

____ 45. Nurse change agents could use this theory to create change in nursing education.

____ 46. Nurse change agents could use this theory to create change in nursing administration.

VI. Foresight

____ 47. The theory helps change agents to foresee possible procedural pitfalls in planning change.

____ 48. The theory helps change agents to foresee possible cultural pitfalls in planning change.

____ 49. The theory suggests ways to deal with possible procedural pitfalls in planning change.

____ 50. The theory suggests ways to deal with possible cultural pitfalls in planning change.

____ 51. The theory helps change agents to foresee immediate resistance to change.

____ 52. The theory helps change agents to foresee long-term resistance to change.

____ 53. The theory helps change agents to foresee the immediate results of adopting the proposed solutions.

____ 54. The theory helps change agents to foresee the long-term results of adopting the proposed solutions.

Scoring: This tool helps you to see how well the change theory fits your specific change situation. As you score the statements, you are able to tell how well the theory meets your change process needs. Overall, the higher the total score (adding up each number for all 54 items = highest total score 216), the better the fit between the change theory and your change situation.

CASE STUDY

Evelyn, a nurse manager of a 47-bed oncology unit in a large teaching hospital in Cincinnati, Ohio, decides to implement a new system of shift reporting because the current system is too lengthy. She first introduces the idea at a staff meeting and discusses several different options as well as the problems with the current system. She discusses the difficulties of providing high quality client care for the first 45 minutes of each shift. Evelyn then opens the meeting for discussion. She encourages both objections and support for each idea. Evelyn elicits volunteers to work on the planned change. After two months, Evelyn asks the task force to report back their findings and propose a new method for the reporting structure for the unit. Individuals are again encouraged to both critique and support the proposal. After this meeting, modifications in the new reporting format are made and the plan is implemented. Evelyn and the task force make a point to reinforce the change with the staff and to provide them with encouragement and support when any difficulties arise.

Case Study Questions

1. Did Evelyn use a change theory? If so, which one?
2. What steps of the change theory do you see in this case study?
3. Why did Evelyn and the task force encourage the staff to raise concerns and verbalize resistance?

LEARNING RESOURCES

Discussion Questions

1. Discuss the similarities and differences of Lippitt's and Havelock's change theories.
2. What is an innovation? Discuss nursing innovations with which you are familiar.
3. Discuss potential emotional responses to change, and describe how you would facilitate the change process when encountering these responses.
4. What are four major changes occurring in the healthcare industry today? What are some strategies to manage these changes effectively?
5. How can resistance positively affect change? What should a leader do when resistance is encountered?

Study Questions

True or False: Circle the correct answer.

T   F   1. Change is inevitable and is necessary for organizational viability.
T   F   2. Resistance can be useful and should be listened to and analyzed.
T   F   3. Lippitt's change theory involves the phases of unfreezing, moving, and refreezing.
T   F   4. Change is a linear process requiring a series of discrete steps.
T   F   5. Resistance most commonly arises because individuals are trying to gain more power.
T   F   6. Changing individual behavior requires considerable time and energy.
T   F   7. Individuals become aware of the need for change when needs are unmet.
T   F   8. Position power can be used effectively to initiate change.
T   F   9. Change occurs in a logical, planned manner.
T   F   10. Too much change is disruptive and can create disorganization in an organization.

SUPPLEMENTAL READINGS

Drucker, P. (1992). *Managing for the future: The 1990s and beyond.* New York: Truman Talley Books/Plume.

McCloskey, J., Maas, M., Huber, D., Kasparek, A., Specht, J., Ramler, C., Watson, C., Blegin, M., Delaney, C., Ellerbe, S., Kelly, K., Mehmert, P., & Clougherty, J. (1994). Nursing management innovations: A need for systematic evaluation. *Nursing Economics, 12*(1), 35-44.

Perlman, D. & Takacs, G. (1990). The 10 stages of change. *Nursing Management, 21*(4), 33-38.

Tiffany, C.R., Cheatham, A.B., Doornbos, D., Loudermelt, L., and Momadi, G.G. (1994). Planned change theory: Survey of nursing periodical literature. *Nursing Management, 25*(7), 54-59.

Chapter 27

Performance Appraisal

STUDY FOCUS

Performance appraisals are important in managing the quality, efficiency, and effectiveness in the provision of nursing services. Consumers and regulatory agencies are looking for assurances that practitioners are competent to provide client services within their scope of practice. One method of evaluating the practice or work of an employee is through annual performance appraisals. A conventional performance appraisal is a systematic standardized evaluation of an employee by a superior for the purpose of evaluating quality, effectiveness, and potential for advancement. Currently, employer evaluation is often complemented by peer and self-evaluation to provide an enhanced description of quality and competence from multiple perspectives. Peer review consists of written or verbal input by those peers who work with the employee being evaluated into the performance appraisal. These are peers who are knowledgeable about the employee's level of performance. The goal of performance appraisals is to improve performance.

Typically, individuals' performances combine their ability and their motivation. Ability is either acquired through learning or innate, and motivation is the willingness and desire to perform work. Employees may become discouraged and lack motivation when it is punishing to complete work, when nonperformance is rewarded, when the quality of performance makes no difference, and when there are barriers to performance. Some components of evaluation are subjective, such as an evaluator's value system and expectations, and these influence the rating of an employee.

The goals of a comprehensive appraisal system include fulfilling the job description requirements, improving on employees' skills, rewarding employee motivation, and matching the right employees with the right job. Evaluations are based on standards. Absolute standards are the evaluator's personal expectations of employees based on values and knowledge. A comparative standard is a measurement system in which employees are compared to one another and

ranked accordingly. The steps in the appraisal process include assessing and evaluating organizational needs, establishing organizational goals with specific time frames, and assessing and evaluating employee progress. In many organizations, performance assessment is continual and aimed at educating employees through coaching; through counseling to improve skills; and through on-going, nonthreatening evaluation.

The job description and performance appraisal tool are documents that employees can use as guides to management's values. Performance appraisals improve performance and communication, reinforce positive behavior, provide rewards, document reasons for termination, and assist individuals with learning needs. Ten research-based principles for performance appraisal are rewarding and developing subordinates, training managers in evaluation, basing evaluation on job descriptions, involving employees in the evaluation, setting mutually agreed upon goals, focusing on problem solving, separating evaluation from counseling, providing administrative support, matching job expectations with evaluation, and generating useful data for administrative decisions.

There are many performance measurement tools to evaluate performance including anecdotal notes, open-ended essays, checklists, rating scales, and behaviorally anchored rating scales. Anecdotal notes are written data about employee performance. Open-ended essays are written descriptions of employee performance. Checklists identify desired behaviors or activities, and rating scales assess each behavior on a numerical rating, usually from 1 to 5. Behaviorally anchored rating scales require the documentation of behaviors as well as a numerical ranking.

Commonly, evaluators err in evaluation. The most common evaluator errors are the halo effect, the recency effect, problem distortion, the sunflower effect, the central tendency effect, the rater temperament effect, and the guessing error. The halo effect occurs when evaluators' rank all categories high when an individual does well in several areas but not all. Recency effect occurs when the evaluator rates the employee based on recent events rather than the full year. Problem distortion is when the evaluator only remembers the problems with an employee's performance. The sunflower effect occurs when evaluators rate everyone high because they are part of a high performance team, and central tendency effect is when the evaluator rates everyone average in order to avoid conflict. Rater temperament effect is when the boss errs on the side of leniency or strictness in evaluation, and guessing errors occur when the evaluator is behind in his work and estimates performance instead of collecting objective data.

LEARNING TOOLS

Activity

Purpose: To practice writing peer evaluations to include specific measurable data.

Scenario: Hillary is a hard-working RN who consistently provides excellent quality care to her assigned clients. She always helps others when her work is completed and has good working relationships with physicians, families, and other healthcare workers. One area Hillary despises is charting. She charts in a cursory, objective style, but does not always document everything that is needed. Rarely does she contribute to the nursing care plan, which necessitates others completing this work. Hillary is active in the Oncology Nursing Society and regularly attends continuing educational offerings. She has joined the unit-based quality improvement committee and contributes valuable information.

Directions: Below you will find a form that you must complete as Hillary's peer evaluator. Remember to make the notations as objective as possible. Descriptions of each category are listed below the client behavior and Likert scale. A Likert scale is used to rank her performance with a range of 1 for outstanding to 5 for unsatisfactory.

When making comments about Hillary's performance, use specific measurable objective data. For example, a comment in the professional development section might read: Hillary has been a member of the unit-based quality improvement committee for four months and attends regularly. Hillary has brought many ideas for improving processes on the unit, such as walking rounds instead of report, flexible hours for employees, and the need to develop procedures for new oncological treatments.

Clinical Behaviors

Client Care   1   2   3   4   5

Refers to client care activities such as personal care, treatments, medication administration, and coordination of care with physicians and other healthcare workers.

Comments:

_____

_____

_____

Team Work   1   2   3   4   5

Works with peers, physicians, clients, and other healthcare workers to maximize positive client outcomes and improve quality.

Comments:

_____

_____

_____

Client Teaching 1   2   3   4   5

Individualizes a teaching plan for each assigned client, documents the teaching, and reports teaching needs during shift report.

Comments:

_____

_____

_____

Committee Participation   1   2   3   4   5

Actively participates in at least one unit-based committee. Contributes to the committee process by chairing a committee, providing information for committee work, or completing the work of the committee.

Comments:

_____

_____

_____

Charting   1   2   3   4   5

Documents timely, accurately, and comprehensively all client care activities, medications, and treatments.

Comments:

_____

_____

_____

Nursing Care Plans   1   2   3   4   5

Initiates care plans for newly admitted clients during the shift of admission, updates, and modifies nursing care plans.

Comments:

_____

_____

_____

Professional Involvement   1   2   3   4   5

Dresses professionally, participates in professional organization activities, attends continuing educational seminars, and provides leadership in unit-based activities.

Comments:

_____

_____

_____

CASE STUDY

Stephanie is a nurse manager of a 75-bed oncology unit in large teaching hospital in Atlanta, Georgia. Stephanie has been a nurse manager at this hospital for fifteen years and has developed a high performance team on her unit. She personally interviews all applicants for her unit and encourages staff participation in the final selection. Stephanie frequently volunteers for pilot projects and is able to garner resources for staff projects. Stephanie finds performance evaluations difficult and has decided to rank everyone the same this year because they all perform so well as a team. She has decided to rank everyone high.

Case Study Questions

1. What type of evaluator error has Stephanie committed?
2. What are some other methods of evaluation that could assist Stephanie to make choices about employee ranking?
3. How could Stephanie use the performance appraisal process to assist the staff to individualize their learning needs as well as to meet organizational objectives?

LEARNING RESOURCES

Discussion Questions

1. What is the purpose of annual performance appraisals, and how should a nurse manager go about collecting objective data?
2. Is objectivity possible in a performance appraisal system? If so, how can a nurse manager make the appraisal process as objective as possible?
3. What are the current trends in annual performance appraisals in regard to who has what kind of input into employee evaluations?
4. In your organization, are employee performance appraisal ratings tied to monetary rewards? Or are the performance appraisal ratings used for self-improvement, and an across the board raise is given to employees? Which system of reward would motivate you?
5. Do you feel comfortable in providing and receiving peer evaluation? Do you find peer evaluation useful in upgrading your skills?

Study Questions

Matching: Write the letter of the correct response in front of each term.

_____ 1. performance appraisal

_____ 2. peer review

_____ 3. absolute standard

_____ 4. comparative standard

_____ 5. anecdotal notes

_____ 6. open-ended essays

_____ 7. checklists

_____ 8. rating scales

_____ 9. behaviorally anchored rating scales

_____ 10. sunflower effect

A. evaluations reference-based with other employee performance

B. list of desired employee behaviors

C. rating everyone high because they are part of a high performing team

D. ratings based on documentation of employee behaviors

E. evaluation based on the manager's own values

F. paragraph descriptions of employee behaviors and performance

G. numerical scores for assessing employee behaviors

H. written records of employee behaviors

I. evaluating the work of others

J. assessing the level of work by an associate

SUPPLEMENTAL READINGS

Keyes, M. (1994). Recognition and reward: A unit-based program. *Nursing Management, 25*(2), 52-54.

Pfeffer, J. & Langton, N. (1993). The effect of wage dispersion on satisfaction, productivity, and working collaboratively. *Administrative Science Quarterly, 38*(3), 382-407.

Chapter 28

Productivity and Costing Out Nursing

STUDY FOCUS

Productivity is key to organizational financial viability. Productivity is the ratio of resources used to provide the service (input) to client outcomes or services (output). The administrative team in healthcare organizations is faced with decreasing reimbursement for services and with capitated payment systems. To compete effectively for market share, healthcare organizations must provide quality services at reasonable costs. Capitated systems require that organizations provide a package of comprehensive services to clients for a fixed fee per head. If healthcare organizations are to survive, they must provide the services effectively and efficiently. Effectiveness is doing the right things correctly to achieve established outcomes. Efficiency is providing the necessary services quickly and inexpensively.

Nurse managers must be cognizant of productivity levels and the cost of nursing services in order to manage a healthcare organization effectively. The term *costing of nursing services* refers to the cost of services or interventions carried out by nurses. Nursing productivity is a combination of nursing care hours and the provision of nursing care services. To increase productivity nurses can provide services with fewer nursing care hours or complete more interventions in a shorter time period. The challenge is to increase productivity, ensure quality, and empower employees to improve processes. Employee productivity can be increased by substituting equipment for labor, improving work methods, removing unproductive practices, and improving human resource management.

Nurse managers must possess refined skills in calculating productivity. Calculating hours per patient day (HPPD) is the oldest nursing productivity index and is imprecise. Other methods include dividing input by output, dividing cost by unit of output, dividing dollars by worked hours, dividing nursing hours worked by the number of hospital client days, and dividing the number of nursing staff by census of client days. When determining productivity, both decision making and tasks must be included in workload calculations. Standards of care, time and motion studies, and job descriptions provide a basis for developing tools to collect workload data.

The cost-effectiveness and cost-benefit models assist in determining productivity. The cost-effectiveness model examines different methods of obtaining desired outcomes. It examines different programs whose objectives vary in order to determine the most productive method of providing services. The cost-benefit model is resource-driven, while the cost-effectiveness model is goal-driven. Productivity measures are complex because measuring nursing care outcomes is controversial. Nursing care and outcomes are not standardized, and a single best method for resource use in nursing interventions is not clearly delineated.

Costing out nursing services is important in order to facilitate nursing's input in public health decisions, health policy, and reimbursement decisions. Costing out nursing services provides data to facilitate comparative productivity measures within and between organizations. Specific costs then can be determined for each nursing intervention and nursing diagnosis, which in turn further establishes a mechanism for determining third party reimbursement. Organizational survival will depend on shrewd management and leadership in controlling costs, in empowering employees to improve and streamline processes, and in procuring resources for promising innovations.

LEARNING TOOLS
Productivity Assessment

Purpose: To practice calculating simple productivity measures, and to understand the importance of productivity in healthcare organizations.

Methods for Calculating Productivity

A. $\dfrac{\text{OUTPUT (dollars)}}{\text{INPUT (work hours)}} = \text{P (productivity)}$

Explanation: Input can include supplies, equipment, labor, and overhead expenses for the building. This simple calculation provides insight into the work hours per revenue generated ratio. Several things must be examined by a nurse manager when she examines her monthly budget reports. Is the unit over-budget in supplies, equipment expenditures, or labor? Are client days high, low, or on-budget? All these factors will impact the amount of profit generated by the unit. Work hours divided by dollars give one quick picture of labor expense to revenue generated.

OR

B. $\dfrac{\text{TOTAL COST}}{\substack{\text{UNIT OF OUTPUT}\\ \text{(client days)}}} = \text{P (productivity)}$

Explanation: The cost of managing the care of clients is based on multiple factors. One factor is the volume of clients for which care is provided. Another is the dollar amount required to provide that care. Try the following set of calculations in order to assess Unit A's productivity. First you need to know that Unit A's fixed cost to operate annually is $300,000 with a variable cost per day of $100 for each of the 6000 client days.

Calculate the cost of each client day by combining the fixed cost and the bariable cost ($ per day x # of client days) to reach the total cost. Then using the formula, divide the total cost by the output (# of client days) to find the total cost per client day. (See the end of the section for answers.)

step one:

step two:

step three:

OR

C. $\dfrac{\text{COST OF DIRECT CARE}}{\text{WORK HOURS}} = \text{P (productivity)}$

Explanation: A cost per direct care hour can be determined by taking the total budgeted cost for the department and dividing it by the total budgeted direct client care hours. The cost per direct care hour is

important because it indicates the average cost of care for a client. The direct care hour cost is usually based on productive (worked) hours.

Try the following set of calculations in order to assess Unit B's productivity. First you need to know that the total budgeted cost for labor for the unit is $600,000, and the total number of direct client care hours are 43,680.

Divide the total budgeted cost for labor by direct client care hours to get the total direct care hour cost.

step one:

OR

D. $\dfrac{\substack{\text{NURSING HOURS}\\ \text{\# OF HOSPITAL}\\ \text{CLIENT DAYS}}}{} = \text{P (productivity)}$

OR

$\dfrac{\substack{\text{NUMBER OF}\\ \text{NURSING STAFF}}}{\text{CENSUS}} = \text{P (productivity)}$

Explanation: The number of hours worked divided by the number of hospital client days reflects the acuity level of clients. This can be compared to budgeted levels of nursing hours per hospital day; from these numbers, the overall productivity level can be assessed.

Another approach is dividing the number of staff by the census or client days. This provides an overall staff to client ratio, which typically stays relatively constant. Deviation from the typical staff/client ratio gives a manager an indication of increased or decreased staff productivity.

Answer to B:

Step one:
6,000 (client days) x $100/day = $600,000

Step two:
$600,000 (variable cost) + $300,000 (fixed cost) = $900,000

Step three:
$\dfrac{\$900,000 \text{ (total cost)}}{6,000 \text{ (client days)}} = \$150$ per client day

Answer to C:

$\dfrac{\$600,000 \text{ (labor costs)}}{43,680 \text{ (direct client care hours)}} = \$13.74$ dollars per direct care hour.

CASE STUDY

Karen, a nurse manager of a 23-bed step-down unit in a medium-size hospital in El Paso, Texas, prides herself on the fact that her unit has the highest quality scores in the hospital. The clinical staff who work on the step-down unit consistently document all nursing interventions and pertinent client data, carry out procedures according to protocol, and go out of their way to facilitate the client's journey to health and wellness. Many physicians use the step-down unit as an example of excellence in client care. The only problem that Karen has is keeping the unit on budget and maintaining a high level of productivity. In comparison to the other units, the step-down unit has a low productivity level and a high budget.

Case Study Questions

1. Is the unit Karen manages efficient?
2. Is the unit Karen manages effective?
3. What would you do if you were the manager? Would you maintain status quo or try to improve productivity?

LEARNING RESOURCES

Discussion Questions

1. What type of activities could help leaders increase employee productivity? What type of activities could help managers increase employee productivity?
2. What is productivity? How do you measure productivity?
3. What are the different types of reimbursement systems in healthcare today?
4. What are some changes that could be made on your unit in order to improve productivity?
5. What is the cost-effectiveness model? What is the cost-benefit model? Give an example of a situation in which you would use each of these models.

Study Questions

True or False: Circle the correct answer.

T   F   1. Productivity is measured by calculating the cost of nursing care multiplied by the unit of output.

T   F   2. Effectiveness is how fast or inexpensive a service is provided.

T   F   3. Efficiency is doing the right things to improve quality.

T   F   4. Costing out nursing services is the actual cost of providing services by nurses.

T   F   5. Time and motion studies are no longer valuable in determining workload requirements.

T   F   6. The cost-benefit model is goal-focused and examines different methods to achieve outcomes.

T   F   7. The cost-effectiveness model is a budgetary model that determines costs and assists managers with determining the proper skill mix for a unit.

T   F   8. Economies of scale refer to the productivity of units.

T   F   9. At the present time, doctors are reimbursed for services provided by nurses.

T   F   10. Nurses are in a prime position in the changing healthcare environment and need only to sit and wait for expanded roles in managed care environments.

SUPPLEMENTAL READINGS

Cleland, V. (1990). *The economics of Nursing.* Norwalk, Ct: Appleton & Lange.

Sengin, K. & Dreisbach, A. (1995). Managing with precision: A budgetary decision support model. *The Journal of Nursing Administration, 25*(2), 33-44.

Chapter 29

Managing a Stressful Environment

STUDY FOCUS

Stress is part of a nurse's everyday work. Stress is a physical, psychosocial, or spiritual response to a stressful event called a stressor. Job or occupational stress is an uncomfortable sensation created by the demands of the job or work of the nurse. Nurses experience stress from many sources. Common stressors include clients who are dying or in pain, emergency treatments, demanding co-workers or clients, family commitments, situations in which personal safety is threatened, downsizing, and restructuring. A classic theory that describes stress and stressors is Seyle's general stress theory. Seyle's theory of stress describes stress as a nonspecific state in which each person responds individually to stressors. Most people respond in a "fight or flight" manner.

When stress is too great on the job, nurses may experience burnout. Burnout is a situation in which individuals, experiencing constant long-term stress, respond with emotional and/or physical exhaustion, decreased productivity, and overdepersonalization. New graduates can also experience stress caused by incongruity between their values of idealism and those of the actual work environment, which is called reality shock. New graduates often become disillusioned and decrease their productivity, change jobs, or return to school for a career change.

Coping effectively with stress and changes in the healthcare environment is essential for a satisfied, healthy, and productive employee. Coping is performing activities in an effort to adapt to the situation. Cognitive appraisal is an individual's assessment of the present stressful situation. Stressors can be internal or external to the nurse. Internal stressors can be the personal conflicts of balancing family, work, and social events. External events can include the work environment. Individuals react differently to stressors. Some may deny the existence of the stressors while others become optimistic that they will handle the stressful occurence. Personal hardiness — a characteristic of commitment, control, and willingness to accept a challenge — has been postulated as being important in handling stress. Those nurses that possess characteristics of hardiness are better able to manage their stress.

Hardy (1978) identified different types of role stress. Role stress occurs when individuals are unclear about their job obligations or they feel their obligations are impossible to meet. Role strain is a subjective feeling of distress arising from a response to outside forces. Role ambiguity is when role expectations are unclear to the nurse. Role conflict is experienced when role expectations are incompatible with each other. Role incongruity occurs when role expectations are incompatible with the professional values of the nurse. Role overload occurs when a nurse cannot possibly complete all assigned activities in the scheduled time frame. Role underload occurs when nurses with advanced training are not able to use their skills to the fullest extent.

Nurses must learn positive coping skills and adaptation strategies to function effectively in their personal and work lives. Individuals who cope effectively reduce their emotional distress, solve their problems, and maintain positive self-esteem. Nurses must carefully examine stressful situations and look out for their best interests. Coping strategies include spending time on recreational activities, creating a personal support network, being involved in a professional association, negotiating or resigning, walking away from problematic situations to reflect, complying when necessary, and modifying rules. Organizations that are attuned to employee well-being organize comprehensive stress management plans to benefit their workers. Strategies to improve well-being include physical activity, nutritional control, environmental control, and support groups.

Nurses have the responsibility for taking care of themselves and others to maximize health and wellness. When nurses become aware of staffing shortages, dangers to personal safety, poor interdepartmental relations, or inadequately designed team situations, they have an obligation to inform their managers of these problematic situations. Being part of a team that takes stressors and turns them into opportunities for innovations or learning boosts employee morale and satisfaction.

LEARNING TOOLS

Self-assessment Stress Test

Purpose: To assess your level of stress.

Directions: Check each event that you have experienced during the past 12 months.

Event	Value	Score	Event	Value	Score
Death of spouse	100	____	Trouble with in-laws	29	____
Divorce	73	____	Outstanding personal achievement	28	____
Marital separation	65	____			
Jail term	63	____	Spouse begins or stops work	26	____
Death of close family friend	63	____			
			Starting or finishing school	26	____
Personal injury or illness	53	____			
			Change in living conditions	25	____
Marriage	50	____			
Fired from work	47	____	Revision of personal habits	24	____
Marital reconciliation	45	____			
Retirement	45	____	Trouble with boss	23	____
Change in family member's health	44	____	Change in work hours conditions	20	____
Pregnancy	40	____	Change in residence	20	____
Sex difficulties	39	____	Change in schools	20	____
Addition to family	39	____	Change in recreational habits	19	____
Business readjustment	39	____			
			Change in church activities	19	____
Change in financial status	38	____			
			Change in social activities	18	____
Death of close friend	37	____			
			Mortgage or loan under $10,000	17	____
Change to different line of work	36	____			
			Change in sleeping habits	16	____
Change in number of marital arguments	35	____			
			Change in number of family gatherings	15	____
Mortgage or loan over $10,000	31	____			
			Change in eating habits	15	____
Foreclosure of mortgage or loan	30	____			
			Vacation	13	____
Change in work responsibilities	29	____	Christmas season	12	____
			Minor violations	11	____
Son or daughter leaving home	29	____			

Total Points _____

Scoring: Add up your score of stress related events which occurred during the last 12 months. If your score falls at 150 points or less you're fairly safe from developing a stress-related illness. If your score falls between 151–299 you have a 50% chance of developing a stress-related illness and if your score is 300 or more you have an 80% chance of developing a stress-related illness.

Reprinted by permission of the publisher from The social readjustment rating scale, Holmes, T.H. & Rahe, R.H, Journal of Psychosomatic Research, vol. 11, pp. 213-218. copyright 1967 by Elsevier Science Inc.

CASE STUDY

Kelsey, a clinical nurse on a 18-bed protective care unit in a community hospital in Rock Springs, Wyoming, has worked for the hospital for twenty years. Kelsey has observed many changes at the hospital, but lately there are several changes occurring at once with restructuring, quality improvement processes, downsizing, and the addition of UAPs. Kelsey has been feeling physically exhausted and depersonalized, and her productivity is declining. Kelsey feels helpless and would like all the changes to stop, so that she could just provide good individualized client care. Lately, co-workers have noticed that Kelsey does the minimum possible to get by and leaves promptly at the stroke of 3:00 P.M. when her shift ends.

Case Study Questions

1. What syndrome is Kelsey experiencing?
2. What is causing her to feel hlepless and to begin to decompensate?
3. What can Kelsey do now to help herself function effectively when providing client care?

LEARNING RESOURCES

Discussion Questions

1. What are effective coping strategies for nurses to use in order to stay healthy and deliver optimal client care?
2. What is occupational or job stress? What causes job stress? How can nurses work effectively when experiencing job stress?
3. What is Seyle's general stress theory? Describe how this theory is applicable in nursing.
4. What is the difference between reality shock and burnout? Describe and give an example of each.
5. How can nurses be proactive and use stress to their benefit? Give an example.

Study Questions

Matching: Write the letter of the correct response in front of each term.

_____ 1. stress
_____ 2. stressor
_____ 3. burnout
_____ 4. reality shock
_____ 5. role incongruity
_____ 6. role ambiguity
_____ 7. hardiness
_____ 8. role overload
_____ 9. role underload
_____ 10. role strain

A. occurs when nurses with advanced training are not able to use their skills to the fullest

B. when a nurse cannot possibly complete all assigned activities in the scheduled time frame

C. when role expectations are incompatible with the professional values of the nurse

D. when role expectations are unclear to the nurse

E. subjective feeling of distress arising from responses to outside forces

F. new graduates experience of incongruity in their values of idealism and the work environment

G. long-term stress resulting in exhaustion or decreased productivity

H. characteristics of commitment, control, and willingness to accept a challenge

I. a stressful event

J. a physical, social, or spiritual response to an event

SUPPLEMENTAL READINGS

Hagenow, N. & McCrea, M. (1994). A mentoring relationship: Two viewpoints. *Nursing Management, 25*(12), 42-43.

Merry, M. & Singer, D. (1994). Healing the healers. *Healthcare Forum Journal, 37*(6), 37-41.

Chapter 30

Health Policy and the Nurse

STUDY FOCUS

Political, social, and economic changes in the United States are creating far reaching changes in healthcare delivery systems. Nurses must clearly articulate what nursing is, what services they provide, and at what costs in order to compete in a competitive healthcare environment. Changes in reimbursement methods, increasing demands for services by consumers, and the competition for market share demand that nurses provide accessible, quality services at reasonable costs. Nursing leadership must be active in legislation for healthcare providers and services. They must also impact policy on reimbursement for nursing services and clearly articulate nursing's role in healthcare delivery. Nurses must be involved in setting policy. Policy is the development of value statements, and setting goals and direction. Nurses must also be involved in politics which involves influencing the allocation of scarce resources by setting health policy. Health policy is the set of public policies that pertain to health and illness. Health policy can be classified as allocative, which means it subsidizes a group, or regulatory, which means it ensures that objectives are met.

Public policy is formulated through governmental activities. The policy-making process occurs in three phases and is generally initiated by a small but powerful group, by a widespread problem that affects a large group, or by the media. The first phase is policy formulation, which involves agenda setting and developing legislation. During policy formulation, much debate and input is generated with special interest groups and other influential leaders either to encourage legislation or to prevent a bill. The second phase is policy implementation, which is when the legislation is implemented. At this phase, the law is vague and the details of implementation must be established. The third phase is policy modification. In this phase changes are made as the legislation is being formulated or during implementation. The legislation frequently is modified based on competing viewpoints from multiple constituents.

Legislation at the federal level must go through a multistage process in order to become law. The process has many steps, in any of which the bill can die, be modified, or approved. The first step is to introduce a legislative proposal, also called a bill. Anyone can have input into the drafting of the bill, but only a member of Congress can sponsor the legislation. The member of Congress who is sponsoring the bill introduces it to his or her chamber where the bill will be numbered and referred to a standing committee. Hearings are then held, and the bill is marked up. The committee reports back to the chamber, and the bill is placed on the legislative agenda and then debated. During this process the bill can stand as is or be amended. The bill will either pass or be defeated. If the bill passes, it goes to the other chamber for a similar process. If both chambers approve the bill, it is sent to the President, who may choose to sign it, veto it (a two-thirds vote of both houses overrides a Presidential veto), or hold it (it will become law within ten days).

Nurses must be politically active to have an impact on their own opportunities and on client welfare in health policy. Nurses can call their legislators; write letters clearly articulating their expectations and positions; join professional organizations to ensure a collective, united voice; support local and state activities; assist during a campaign for a state representative; vote, and rally others to vote; form and participate in a protest rally; and help draft legislation. Another important activity is to assist in writing professional position papers through the American Nurses' Association and to conduct and share essential nursing research studies with legislators that support key issues. Nurses can stay abreast of current legislative activities by reading the newsletters of professional organizations and professional journals, reading newspapers, watching news on the television, and networking with colleagues. Major changes are occurring in healthcare. Nurses must be instrumental in formulating legislation to ensure nursing's position in the healthcare delivery system.

LEARNING TOOLS

Self-assessment

Purpose: To become aware of the strategies for nurses to become politically active in improving health policy

Introduction: There are many activities that you can engage in to become politically active and support a specific health policy. One strategy is to call your legislators and discuss the importance of a bill or issue. You can provide specific details about why it is important and how it will benefit the public. For example, if the issue is providing reimbursement for nurse practitioners, essential points to discuss are the importance of eliminating financial barriers and improving access to care for families in your state. You can also provide references from nursing research articles about the increased quality, access, and decreased costs for care provided by nurse practitioners to support your position. Additional strategies to support nurse practitioners are refering clients to them, personally seeking care from them, and talking to the community about the important role nurse practitioners play in the healthcare delivery system.

Follow-up with the legislator by providing a written letter addressing specific points, support for laws on the reimbursement of nurse practitioners and reasons why this is important. Include any resources that might help support your case for expanded reimbursement for nurse practitioners.

Directions: Identify an issue that you are concerned about and would like to see changed or supported by your legislator. Call the legislator, and discuss the issue with them. Then send a follow-up letter detailing your position, and include any documents of support. You will find a letter provided, showing you the components to include in the letter to your legislator. It is important to send a typed letter.

Date

Name
Title
Address

To: Name

In this section clearly identify what you expect of the legislator. Example: I would like you to support legislation and policies to remove barriers to equitable reimbursement for nurses in (identify your state).

Describe why it is important for your legislator to support your issue. Example: A nurse practitioner is a registered nurse who has successfully completed a graduate program in a nursing specialty and functions in an expanded practice role. These nurses are able to provide primary care to communities, increasing accessible, affordable, quality healthcare.

At this point, it is useful to cite statistics or research about the cost, quality, or outcomes nurse practitioners are able to provide. Example: I have enclosed two studies that demonstrate the benefits for the clients of nurse practitioners who provide care. These studies show that the cost of care to clients is decreased, risk factors are identified, and lifestyle modifications are implemented to decrease detrimental effects on health.

In this section summarize your request, restate what you expect, and close the letter. Example: I look forward to your support for equitable reimbursement for nurses in (state). Nurse practitioners increase access to care and provide high quality holistic healthcare at a reasonable cost.

Sincerely,

Name, Credentials

CASE STUDY

Jason is an RN on a 45-bed obstetric unit in a large teaching hospital in Birmingham, Alabama. Jason is a primary nurse for both mothers and infants. He always completes a nursing care assessment and then follows up by making a telephone call to track the client's progress. Jason has a population of clients who are indigent and frequently request additional teaching on parent/child care activities. Jason is concerned that the mothers do not have the support or information available to them to provide the best possible care for their infants. Jason conducted a research study on a subset of his clients and divided the group into two. One group received home visits and assistance with nutritional needs, and the other only received a follow-up questionnaire and a single visit to evaluate the parent/child interaction. Jason noticed a marked improvement in the infants in the first group. The infants were more responsive, were more advanced in their activity level, and were all within normal limits for weight gain. The infants in the other group, however, were less active, less responsive, and 30% were underweight for their age. Jason decides that he needs to find a way to support mothers who needs assistance. He becomes politically active to garner support for his interventions.

Case Study Questions

1. What should Jason do to garner support for his ideas?
2. How can his research assist to support his ideas?
3. How long a process is it to change or implement a new program with state or federal moneys?

LEARNING RESOURCES

Discussion Quesions

1. What changes in the delivery of healthcare to clients have occured as a result of the national healthcare reform initiatives in the United States?
2. What can nurses do to become politically active and have a strong voice in healthcare policy?
3. In what phases of the policy-making process can nurses initiate changes to improve the public's health?
4. Does nursing have a strong special interest group in Washington?
5. Describe the multistage process of how a bill becomes law and identify strategies nurses can use to initiate or enhance legislation.

Study Questions

True or False: Circle the correct answer.

T	F	1. The three phases of policy making are policy formulation, policy implementation, and policy modification.
T	F	2. Policy issues are raised only when they impact the small, but powerful groups in the United States.
T	F	3. Policy making is a very analytical process based solely on objective data.
T	F	4. Nursing research should be an important component of the policy making process.
T	F	5. Politics is the same thing as power.
T	F	6. An allocative health policy ensures that objectives are met.
T	F	7. Ethical decisions should remain separate and not be discussed when public policy is set.
T	F	8. A white paper is usually drafted by a professional organization to clearly define their position on a specific topic.
T	F	9. Politics is the attempt to influence the allocation of scarce resources.
T	F	10. The terms public policy and health policy can be used interchangeably.

SUPPLEMENTAL READINGS

Coopers & Lybrand. (1994). Healthcare reform: Innovations at the state level. *Nursing Management, 25*(4), 30-35, 38-40, 42.

Johnson, S. (1994). GME financing: A well-kept secret. *Nursing Management, 25*(4), 43-46.

Chapter 31

Career Development

STUDY FOCUS

Nurses enter the profession of nursing for many reasons. Some enter to help people, others for job security, and still others were influenced by a role model. Nurses may view their work as a job or a career. A job is a specific position that one fills for a specific amount of pay, whereas a career is a personal and professional plan comprised of a series of positions to meet a long-term goal. Career commitment is an individual's motivation and attitude to work in a professional role. Nurses assesses their personal and professional goals in relation to their work, themselves, and family obligations when determining a career trajectory or professional path. Examining adult life stages when assessing an individual's career trajectory assists in understanding choices throughout the life span in relation to developmental growth and task accomplishment. Early in an individual's career, between the ages of 18 and 22, one experiences an exploration phase; between 46 and 53 one balances one's life, and after the age of 70 one does what one is able to. An individual's career choice is influenced by the work, personal and family needs, and roles in one's life.

Individuals who view nursing as a profession need to plan their career and then follow it up with periodic self-analysis to examine their needs and goals. Self-assessments are important at annual intervals in order to see progress toward personal and professional goals and again at times of decision when choices must be made about changing positions, returning for advanced education, taking a certification exam, or moving to a new location.

Career anchors are personal needs and skills that help to explain individual values in career choices. Friss (1989) identified eight career anchors which are service, managerial competence, autonomy, technical-functional competence, security, identity, variety, and creativity. Nurses tend to especially value the three primary anchors of technical-functional competence, security, and identity. An advantage for individuals pursuing a nursing career is the variety of roles available and the multiple part-time opportunities for employment. Many nurses are keenly aware of the social, political, and economic environment that has an impact on opportunities within the profession of nursing, as well as the timing of personal and family goals and demands.

Career planning is essential to meeting professional goals. Career planning is most effective when started early in an individual's career. Self-assessment is the cornerstone of career planning, and finding a supportive mentor is useful to advance your career. Vogel (1990) identified career planning as a lifelong process linked to each person's values, lifestyles, goals, and workstyle. Vogel (1990) identified six stages of career development which include self-analysis, career analysis, integrating, planning, implementing, and evaluating. A written plan is beneficial in formulating your personal and professional goals and your plan should be reevaluated annually. To meet your professional goals, you must be aware of environmental changes, set goals, plan activities to enhance your career, and anticipate future trends in order to attain additional education or certification. Then you can capitalize on the changing healthcare environment. Methods for staying informed of healthcare changes include reading professional journals, reading about current events in the national news, joining the American Nurses' Association, networking, and helping with political campaigns.

Benner's (1982) work describes five levels of proficiency that a nurse progresses through to mastery of content and skill. The five levels are novice, advanced beginner, competent, proficient, and expert. Experience and competence are gained over time and require practice and education. Individuals adjust to the work environment and personal and professional demands while gaining expertise. New graduates are commonly in the novice stage of proficiency, and during the transition from school to work, frequently experience reality shock. Reality shock is when a new nurse faces the challenge of implementing the ideal within a constrained work environment. During this period she/he may become disenchanted. Kramer (1974) identifies the honeymoon, shock, recovery, and resolution of conflict as phases of reality shock.

Nurses who choose a career trajectory must be their own advocate for advancement and identify learning opportunities essential for their chosen career path. Marketing yourself is important. Finding a mentor, networking, developing and then assessing your career trajectory, and embarking on advanced preparation, certifications, or specialized training may all be necessary to accomplish your goals. Opportunities in healthcare continually change and keeping abreast of the trends will assist you with career planning. Today, changes in hospital redesign and reengineering are decreasing the number of RNs and limiting the clinical nurse specialist's role. Opportunities are emerging in the areas of primary care and advanced nursing practice. Certification in advanced practice provides recognition by the public of a nurse's specialized area of practice.

LEARNING TOOLS

Self-assessment

Purpose: To assist you in developing a career trajectory, and to develop a cover letter and resume to market your special skills and abilities.

Career Trajectory

Introduction: To successfully plan a career, you need to take time to assess your personal and professional goals in order to develop a meaningful, efficient, and rewarding career trajectory. Once you identify your specific goals, you will be able to determine what resources, education, and experience are essential for you to meet your career goals.

Directions: Conduct a self-assessment of your personal and professional goals. Determine timelines for when you would like certain goals met. You may choose to look at early, middle, and late career and life time goal intervals. Below, a few categories are listed in which you might identify goals. List those goals that you would like to complete in each time period. Form your goals, then fill in the resource category with what you must do to attain your desired goal. For example, if your goal is to be a nurse practitioner, you must pursue advanced education and that would be put into the resource column.

	Early	Middle	Late	Resources
Career Goals				
Lifestyle Goals				
(Personal/Family)				
Financial Goals				
(Living & Retirement)				

Summary: Annually complete a self-assessment to determine at what point you are meeting your goals and what activities you need to engage in to accomplish them.

Cover Letter

Directions: It is important to write a professional cover letter when applying for a position. Even if you choose to deliver the letter and resumé in person, it provides a snapshot of how you present yourself and leaves a strong impression with the recruiter and interview committee. The letter should be clearly written, typed on bond paper, and grammatically correct. Below a sample cover letter is provided for your review. Take the time to develop your own cover letter based on the position(s) you are interested in obtaining. Make sure you get the correct title and spelling of the recruiter's name.

3195 Hanna Ave.
Detroit, MI 68941

January 21, 1996

Phyllis Jones, R.N., M.S.N.
Nurse Recruiter
Cedarville Hospital
719 South Haven
Detroit, MI 68941

Dear Mrs. Jones:

I would like to apply for a position in the six-month graduate nursing internship program for new graduates at Cedarville Hospital that Miss Jason discussed during her visit to Mercy University. Upon graduation with a baccalaureate nursing degree on April 14, 1996, I will be available to begin employment immediately.

Miss Jason's description of Cedarville Hospital as a comprehensive medical center serving the southwestern Detroit community convinced me that the graduate nursing internship is an ideal learning opportunity. I have had two clinical internships on the medical and surgical units at Cedarville Hospital and have been impressed by the high quality care provided by the professional nursing staff. I am interested in joining your professional nursing team.

I am available on Tuesdays and Fridays for an interview. Please let me know if it is convenient for you to meet with me on these days. My telephone number is (313) 687-1519.

I am looking forward t meeting with you and discussing the graduate internship program.

Sincerely,

Sharon Smith

Resumé

Directions: It is important to develop a clear, concise, accurate resumé to convey your work experience, education, and achievements. It is important to devise a simple, but clear format for your resumé. Your resumé should be typed, free from spelling and grammatical errors, and printed on high quality bond paper. Gaps between employment dates need to be explained. A brief description of your employment experience is helpful to highlight key performance areas. A sample resumé follows for your review. Take the time to create a resumé for yourself. This document highlights and markets your abilities. Take the time to make a sharp, professional, accurate resumé. It is important that your resumé stands out among the others and captures the recruiter's attention.

Meghan Sjots
220 South Appleville Drive
Hudsonville, MI 49604
(616) 245-7894

Objective:	To work as a staff nurse on a medical-surgical unit
Education:	B.S.N., Grand Valley State University, Allendale, Michigan, May 1996.
Experience: May 1995- Present	Intern, Butterworth Hospital, Grand Rapids, Michigan
	Assisted registered nurses in providing direct client care — assisted with feeding clients, bathing, taking vital signs, calculating intake and output, positioning, and reporting. Certified in CPR.
May 1994 - May 1995	Volunteer, Butterworth Hospital, Grand Rapids, Michigan
	Coordinated recreation activities for the medical-surgical unit. Transported clients for testing and discharge.
Licensure:	Schedule to sit for the NCLEX in Grand Rapids, Michigan on June 20, 1996.
Professional Organizations:	Michigan Association of Nursing Students
Honors:	Dean's Honor Roll 1992-1996 Kappa Epsilon, Chapter of Sigma Theta Tau Butterworth Hospital Volunteer Award
References:	Available upon request

These references are only provided as a guide of what to submit when you are asked for them.

Julie Brown, R.N., B.S.N.
Nurse Manager Medical-Surgical
Butterworth Hospital
1 Spillwood Avenue
Grand Rapids, Michigan 49580
(616) 791-3456

Mrs. Welch
Volunteer Manager
Butterworth Hospital
1 Spillwood Avenue
Grand Rapids, Michigan 49580
(616) 791-3467

Keverin James, R.N., Ph.D.
Associate Professor of Nursing
Grand Valley State University
1 Campus Drive
Allendale, Michigan 49401
(616) 895-3558

CASE STUDY

Janice is a new graduate who will be graduating from Grand Valley State University with her baccalaureate degree in May 1996. Janice will be interviewing for her first professional nursing position. She has taken the time to develop a professional quality cover letter and resumé. She has researched the available nursing positions in her community and in the surrounding areas. Janice has applied for several positions because of the tight labor market in her area. She is offered two positions — a community health nursing position where she will be a case manager making home visits and helping to coordinate care for a group of families, and a clinical nurse position on a 45-bed medical-surgical unit.

Case Study Questions

1. How should Janice determine which is the best position for her?
2. How does Janice's career trajectory help her make the best decision for her personal and professional goals?
3. Janice has decided that her long-term goal is to become an advanced practice nurse. What is an advanced practice nurse, and how does this plan fit into her present dilemma of which job she should accept?

LEARNING RESOURCES

Discussion Questions

1. How do adult developmental stages relate to career plans and goals?
2. What is advanced practice nursing and how does it relate to nursing careers and career planning?
3. How do healthcare reform issues affect nursing care planning?
4. What are the stages of career planning?
5. What are the benefits of career planning?

Study Questions

True or False: Circle the correct answer.

T   F   1. The most important factor to consider when evaluating job possibilities is the financial remuneration and benefits offered.

T   F   2. Career trajectories provide direction as to what resources, experience, and education are needed.

T   F   3. The career anchors of managerial competence, service, and identity are most representative of nursing.

T   F   4. It is important to stay abreast of changing trends in healthcare as new options may become available in nursing practice.

T   F   5. Career planning is a quick, easy-to-do process that requires little time, but has a big pay off.

T   F   6. Advanced practice nursing refers only to nurse practitioners who are in independent practices in rural areas.

T   F   7. Career plans or trajectories must take into consideration personal, family, and work-related needs for a successful outcome.

T   F   8. A nurse's proficiency level begins with novice and progresses through proficiency, advanced beginner, expert, and then to competence.

T   F   9. Midcareer factors include promotions, job changes, and family and personal obligations.

T   F   10. Nurses should always be aware of their professional image and market themselves as a career development strategy.

SUPPLEMENTAL READINGS

Archibald, P. & Brainbridge, D. (1994). Capacity and competence: Nurse credentialing and privileging. *Nursing Management, 25*(4), 49-51, 54-56.

Benner, P. (1982). From novice to expert. *American Journal of Nursing, 82*(3), 402-407.

Friss, L. (1989). Strategic managment of nurses: A policy-oriented approach. Owings Mills, MD: National Health Publishing.

Keane, A. & Richmond, T. (1993). Tertiary nurse practitioners. *Image, 25*(4), 281-284.

Kramer, M. (1974). *Reality shock: Why nurses leave nursing.* St. Louis: Mosby.

Vogel, G. (1990). Career development: An integrated process. *Holistic Nursing Practice, 4*(4), 46-53.

Answers to Study Questions

Chapter 1

True and False
1. T
2. T
3. F
4. T
5. F
6. F
7. F
8. T
9. F
10. F

Chapter 2

Matching
1. D
2. E
3. B
4. C
5. F
6. A

True and False
1. T
2. F
3. T
4. F

Chapter 3

Matching
1. G
2. A
3. F
4. H
5. B
6. E
7. C
8. D

Chapter 4

Fill in the Blank
1. autocratic — direct leadership is needed.
2. democratic — direction is needed through facilitation and coordination
3. democratic or laissez-faire approach — to provide direction, but allow group leadership and facilitate team work.

True and False
1. T
2. F
3. F
4. T
5. T
6. F
7. F

Chapter 5

True and False
1. F
2. F
3. T
4. T
5. F
6. T
7. F
8. T
9. F
10. T

Chapter 6

Matching
1. G
2. C
3. E
4. F
5. D
6. B
7. A

True and False
1. T
2. F
3. F

Chapter 7

True and False
1. F
2. T
3. T
4. F
5. T
6. T
7. F
8. F
9. F
10. F

Chapter 8

True and False
1. T
2. F
3. F
4. F
5. T
6. F
7. T
8. F
9. T
10. F

Chapter 9

Matching
1. E
2. F
3. G
4. D
5. H
6. I
7. J
8. C
9. B
10. A

Chapter 10

Multiple Choice
1. B
2. D
3. C
4. D
5. A

Chapter 11

True and False
1. T
2. F
3. F
4. T
5. F
6. T
7. F
8. T
9. T
10. F

Chapter 12

Matching
1. I
2. C
3. D
4. E
5. F
6. A
7. B
8. J
9. G
10. H

Chapter 13

Matching
1. I
2. H
3. J
4. G
5. F
6. E
7. D
8. C
9. B
10. A

Chapter 14

True and False
1. F
2. F
3. T
4. F
5. F
6. T
7. T
8. T
9. F
10. F

Chapter 15

Matching
1. J
2. I
3. H
4. G
5. F
6. B
7. D
8. E
9. C
10. A

Chapter 16

Matching
1. J
2. I
3. E
4. D
5. C
6. B
7. F

8. A
9. H
10. G

Chapter 17

True and False
1. T
2. F
3. T
4. F
5. F
6. F
7. T
8. T
9. F
10. T

Chapter 18

True and False
1. F
2. F
3. F
4. F
5. F
6. F
7. F
8. T
9. T
10. T

Chapter 19

Matching
1. G
2. H
3. I
4. D
5. A
6. J
7. B
8. C
9. F
10. E

Chapter 20

Matching
1. D
2. C
3. J
4. H

5. I
6. A
7. B
8. E
9. G
10. F

Chapter 21
True and False
1. F
2. T
3. F
4. F
5. T
6. T
7. T
8. F
9. T
10. F

Chapter 22
Matching
1. I
2. J
3. F
4. E
5. H
6. A
7. B
8. G
9. C
10. D

Chapter 23
True and False
1. F
2. F
3. T
4. T
5. F
6. F
7. T
8. F
9. F
10. T

Chapter 24
Matching
1. E
2. C
3. A
4. B
5. D
6. F
7. H
8. G

Chapter 25
True and False
1. F
2. F
3. T
4. F
5. F
6. F
7. F
8. T
9. T
10. F

Chapter 26
True and False
1. T
2. T
3. F
4. F
5. F
6. T
7. T
8. T
9. F
10. T

Chapter 27
Matching
1. I
2. J
3. E
4. A
5. H
6. F
7. B
8. G
9. D
10. C

Chapter 28
True and False
1. F
2. F
3. F
4. T
5. F
6. F
7. F
8. F
9. T
10. F

Chapter 29
Matching
1. J
2. I
3. G
4. F
5. C
6. D
7. H
8. B
9. A
10. E

Chapter 30
True and False
1. T
2. F
3. F
4. T
5. F
6. F
7. F
8. T
9. T
10. F

Chapter 31
True and False
1. F
2. T
3. F
4. T
5. F
6. F
7. T
8. F
9. T
10. T